One Leg in the Grave Revisited

The miracle of the transplantation of the black leg
by the saints Cosmas and Damian

One Leg in the Grave Revisited

The miracle of the transplantation of the black leg by the saints Cosmas and Damian

Edited by
Kees Zimmerman

With contributions by
Carmen Fracchia,
Jan de Jong,
Catrien Santing

Barkhuis
Groningen
2013

Cover illustration:
illustration in manuscript, Legenda Aurea, end 13th century , HM 3027 fol. 132r (detail).
Henry E. Huntington Library, San Marino (U.S.A.).

Book cover design:
Nynke Tiekstra, ColtsfootMedia, Noordwolde, the Netherlands
Book interior design and typesetting:
Nynke Tiekstra, ColtsfootMedia, Noordwolde, the Netherlands

This publication could not have been achieved without the support of:

U.M.C.G. Groningen, the Netherlands, Department of Transplantation and Organ Donation.

O.I.M. Assen, the Netherlands.

Chios Pharmacy Museum, Greece, www.pharmacymuseum.gr.

Ministerio de Ciencia e Innovación, Spain.
Proyect HAR2010-15970 from the Plan Nacional de Investigación.
Title: "Voces y Ausencias: Esclavitud negroafricana
y abolicionismo en España (siglos XVI al XIX)".

ISBN/EAN: 9789491431234

Contents

Illustrations

Illustrations (general)

Illustrations of the miracle of the transplantation:

Early representations (before 16th century)

Modern representations (20th and 21rst century)

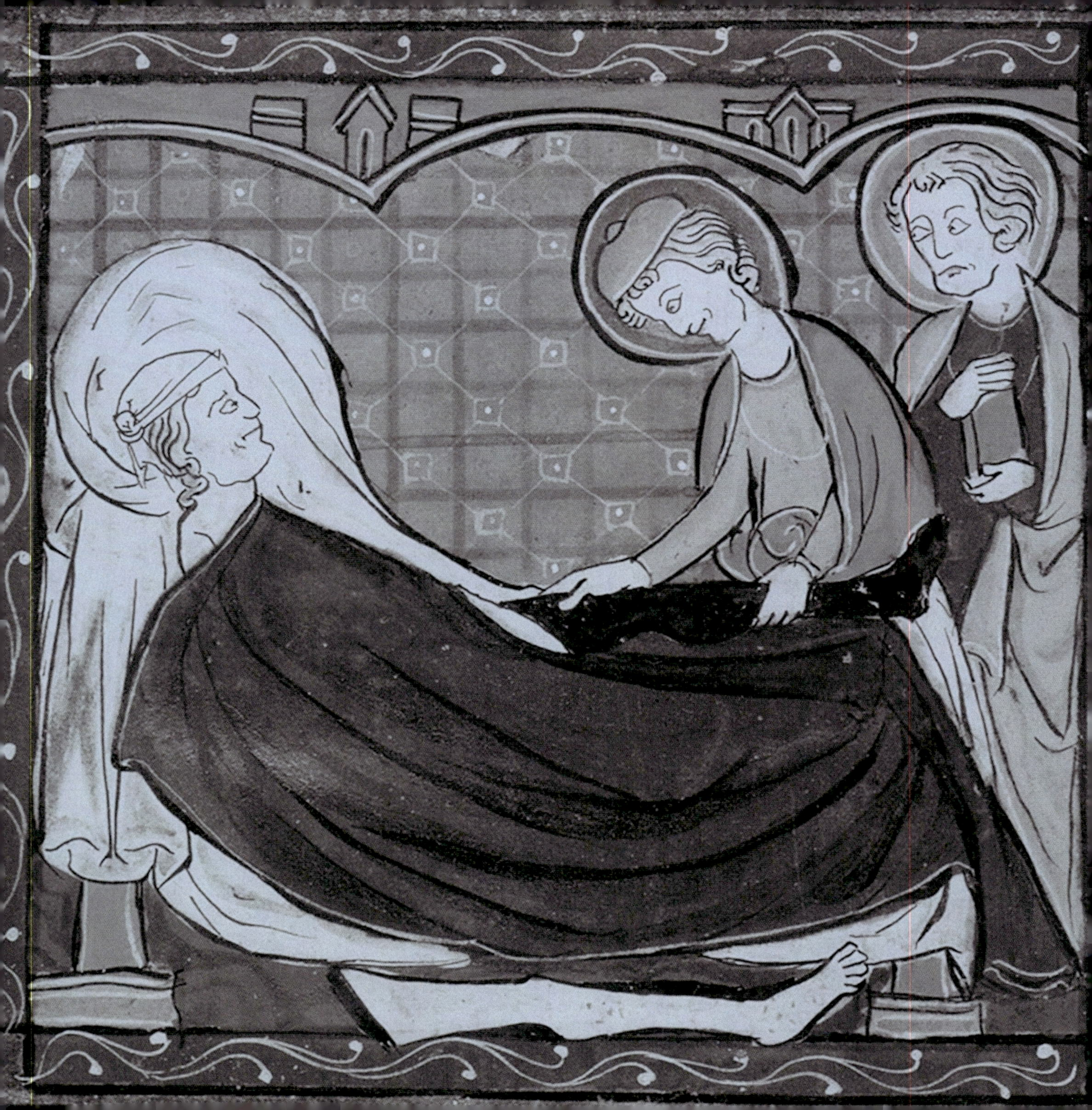

Introduction

Kees Wouter Zimmerman

The life, the suffering and death of saints Cosmas and Damian are described in the *Legenda Aurea*. A number of miracles performed by them is recorded there as well.

The work was written in 1265 by Jacob de Voragine, archbishop of Genua. Before becoming a bishop he already collected accounts of saints' lives, that is during the period that he was a teacher and prior in the Dominican monastery there. The Legenda Aurea is a collection of stories of saints' lives and church festivals, arranged according to the clerical year and mostly compiled and edited from existing and sometimes ancient Greek and Latin texts. The book was initially intended as a reference work for clerics of the Dominican order, who used the legends to embellish their sermons. However, the book was such an unexpected success that it was translated into all Western European vernaculars in the course of the fourteenth century. Before that time legends about the saints were mainly passed on orally. The *Legenda Aurea*, originally entitled Legenda Sanctorum, has become an extensive work. The histories of well over 200 saints have been recorded. One of the saints' stories in Jacob the Voragine's *Legenda Aurea* is that of saints Cosmas and Damian. Probably this legend goes back (partly) to ancient Greek and Latin texts.

Cosmas and Damian were born in the third century AD. They were twin brothers from the town of Aegea. In the Middle Ages the town was called Lajazzo, at present it is called Ayaș, a town in the district of Yumurtalik in the province of Adana in Turkey, located east of the mouth of the Ceyhan River. At the time the district was called Cilicia and it was a province of the Roman Empire. Cosmas and Damian were Christians and were instructed in medicine by the Holy Ghost. Entirely in the spirit of the age they did not want to be rewarded for their medical activities. To this they owe their epithet of *anargyri* (Greek: ἀνάργυροι = without silver money). Many cures performed by them during their lifetime were recorded, among them Palladia's recovery. Palladia was a lady who was ill and who had in vain spent a fortune on doctors. At last she turned to Cosmas and Damian. With their help she recovered completely. By way of thanks she wanted to give Damian a modest gift as a present. At first Damian refused, because as a principle they did not accept any compensation for their medical actions. Yet in order not to insult Palladia he accepted the present in the end. Cosmas was so disgruntled at Damian having accepted a gift that he informed him that he did not want to share the grave with him after his death. The following day the dispute was settled. The only witness of their reconciliation was a camel.

During their life Cosmas and Damian cured both humans and animals. They also performed miracles. When Lysias, the proconsul of Cilicia, heard about the miraculous cures that these Christians, these saints, performed, he had Cosmas and Damian, together with their three brothers, Antimus, Leontius and Euprepius, come and see him. When Lysias ordered them to bring a sacrifice to the Roman gods they refused. Whereupon the five brothers were tortured: in chains they were thrown into the sea but an angel landed the five of them safely ashore. 'Teach me your magic tricks', Lysias said 'and I will be your disciple in the name of the god Adrianus'. Hardly had he said this when two devils appeared and slapped his face. As a consequence the five brothers were then condemned to death. On the funeral pyre Cosmas and Damian remained unscathed, while the onlookers were indeed burnt alive. Next they were crucified and stoned. In the air the stones and arrows turned in the direction of the throwers and wounded them. Cosmas and Damian and their brothers remained unscathed. Finally the five brothers were beheaded. When they were about to be buried, the bystanders remembered the dispute that Cosmas and Damian had about Palladia's gift and had a separate grave dug for Cosmas. Upon this, the camel appeared that had been present when Cosmas and Damian were reconciled. In a human voice the camel said that the past dispute had long been settled and that the five brothers could therefore share the grave, whereupon Cosmas could be also interred in the grave of his four brothers. They died a martyr's death in 287 AD during the reign of the emperor Diocletian.

One of the miracles they posthumously performed in the 6th century AD is generally known. Cosmas and Damian may well owe their fame to this miracle. In Rome Pope Felix had an early Christian temple rebuilt into a church dedicated to Cosmas and Damian. This church employed a pious verger who suffered from a leg affected by cancer. One night in his sleep this verger was visited by Cosmas and Damian. They amputated his leg and replaced it by the leg of a Moor who had just died. The verger woke up, looked at his leg assisted by the light of a candle and to his joy saw that his leg was cured. The transplanted leg was black. The deceased Moor had received the diseased leg. The verger's friends, who did not believe that a miracle had taken place, went to the cemetery of San Pietro in Vincoli where the deceased Moor had been buried and were surprised when they saw that he had received the diseased leg at the precise spot where the black leg had been amputated.

It is only in the version of the miracle in the *Legenda Aurea* that a **black** leg is mentioned.

In the Greek version this miracle takes place in Palestine, and it is not a posthumous miracle. The man with the ulcerated leg lives in the region of Sebastia, and the saints replace his leg with the leg of a recently deceased man. Nowhere is there mention of a black person. The Greek legend goes as follows:

> … the angel Raphael came, and told them: “Go to the temple of the holy martyr, the head of the community. A man is buried there. Go to his grave. For he is lying there for four days. Take his right leg from him and place it on the person who has the diseased leg, in order to help him… And they went and cut off the right leg of the buried man. And they also cut off, at the knee, the ulcerous leg of the man, and attached to him the leg of the buried man, calling upon the name of the Father, the Son, and the Holy Spirit. And as soon as the Holy Trinity was mentioned, the man was found healthy, and the saints, seeing this, praised the Lord. And then they went and brought the leg of the man who had the ulcer to the person who was buried, calling upon the Father, the Son, and the Holy Spirit. And just like he had been with his legs before, so he was found with the leg attached.
> … And he went home in great joy. His neighbours and acquaintances did not believe that his leg had been cut off, until the moment that they went to the grave and saw the leg. Then they believed that it was true what he had told them, and they all glorified God who gave such healing to those who place their hope in God. Glory to Him from eternity to eternity. Amen.”

In our time, in which organ transplants have become commonplace, it is not strange to ponder the transplant of limbs. If we situate transplanting a complete leg in the period in which this was recorded and depicted we discuss something utterly impossible. Stitching on limbs is also familiar in the performances of other saints. For example we know the story of the cut-off hand that is stitched on again by Saint John of Damascus. However, this seems nothing compared to the exchange of a complete leg by a different one. In the present time we have a far too modern and surgical view of such an event. Putting a limb back on takes place in any major hospital across the world. But the transplantation of a limb which results in a completely functioning arm or leg has never been successfully accomplished. It will also take some time before this can be accomplished and lead to a functional extremity. In order to achieve this a number of problems have to be overcome. Surgically connecting the various structures of the donor specimen to that of the receiver is not the greatest problem. Connecting structures such as arteries and nerve fascicles has become possible at microscopic level. With re-implants a certain functionality is achieved, but the original situation is seldom arrived at. However, the result is such that the presence of the re-implanted extremity is clearly to be preferred to its absence. With transplants an additional problem occurs, viz. its rejection by the body. This may be partly avoided by administering medicines, but this influences the recovery, and thus eventually also the functionality of the re-implanted limb. Another harmful effect is the necessity of lifelong administration of these drugs. As it happens they have harmful side effects for the entire body. In transplanting vital organs such as kidneys, liver, heart and lungs we are compelled to take these for granted. With a non-vital organ such as a leg, treatment with a prosthesis still beats treatment with a transplant. Of course this is also because prosthesis have greatly improved over the past few years. However, it is obvious that in future limbs will be transplanted. It is also evident that in doing so medicines will be needed to influence the human defense system.

The Greeks in classical antiquity already knew that in order to transplant a limb medicines were needed in addition to surgery. In Diodorus Siculus Iambulus's voyage to a utopian island is being described. Among other things Iambulus mentions a particular species of turtles living there. With the blood of these turtles it is possible to successfully stitch on lost limbs. The 'ointment' used by Cosmas and Damian in their miraculous cure obviously has the same curative effect as Iambulus's turtle blood. In judging the execution of the miracle by Cosmas and Damian we should therefore imagine ourselves back in the period in which it occurs. At that time stitching on a limb of one's own was equally as impossible as stitching on another person's limb. The replacement of a diseased leg by a healthy black one by Cosmas and Damian should be considered a miracle cure, a variation on stitching on a severed hand. As 'proof' of the exchange of limbs the Moor is provided with the verger's severed leg. The underlying idea may be that one cannot send the Moor to the great beyond with only one leg. A modern surgeon will refrain from returning the severed leg to the donor. This leads to the conclusion that any similarity with present-day transplant surgery is out of the question. However, the story appealed to people, for it was invented, passed on, recorded and extensively portrayed in art.

It was in 1987 that I first saw a painting portraying this miracle of transplanting the black leg. It is a panel by Sano di Pietro in the Pinacotheca Nazionale in Siena (Ill. 13 page 62). It is a splendidly simple representation of the miracle. It emanates peace and quiet. Cosmas and Damian are standing next to bed of the verger who receives the black leg. During the 'operation' the verger is asleep, there is no trace of any pain. No blood flows and surgical instruments are absent. Sano di Pietro has painted a miracle as one imagines a miracle to be. After having seen this painting the representation of the miracle so fascinated me that I continued my search. It was not long before I had collected a dozen pictures. What I discovered until then were illustrations of the most familiar works on this subject. In reading about the lives of saints Cosmas and Damian I regularly came across the names of Marie Louise David-Danel and Pierre Julien. The art historian Marie Louise David-Danel had taken her Ph. D. on the iconography of Cosmas and Damian in Lille in 1958. Pierre Julien, a Parisian pharmacist, was a collector of anything to do with Cosmas and Damian. Illustrations of the miracle of the black leg described in Marie Louise David-Danel's thesis were the starting point for my first searches. I visited almost all of the works mentioned by her and photographed them. Pierre Julien drew my attention to some paintings still missing. Most of those I visited as well. Photos of them were added to my collection. I met both Marie Louise David-Danel and Pierre Julien, at first by exchanging letters, afterwards by visiting the two of them, one in Northern France, the other in Paris. Meanwhile, both unfortunately have died. By contacts with them over the years I received information about missing illustrations of the miracle of the black leg. Apart from them I have met many more people interested in this subject in the past few years. By some of them I was also tipped about any sites with illustrations of the miracle. Things went so far that many holidays that my wife Maaike and I planned took us to churches and museums where supposedly illustrations were to be found. In this way I had collected forty illustrations in 1998. This resulted in the publication of the book 'One Leg in the Grave'. It was published on the occasion of the World Congress ISPO (International Society for Prosthetics and Orthotics) held in Amsterdam in 1998. This book was sold out a couple of years ago, but the number of illustrations I collected kept increasing.

Meanwhile I have collected more than eighty illustrations of the miracle. On most of them it is obvious that the artist wanted to portray the miracle. We see Cosmas and Damian busy at work with the transplant, the transplanted -mostly black- leg being distinctly represented. In some works of art this is less evident. They concern works that are generally regarded as representing the miracle of the transplanted leg. Apparently in those cases it is not always necessary to portray the transplanted (black) leg as well. For example, we see a patient lying in bed, both legs hidden from view, and Cosmas and Damian standing around the bed. The illustration with Cosmas and Damian next to the bed is not always connected with the transplant miracle, since the curing of a diseased person may also be depicted. In a few instances we know that, as in the illustration in a Greek manuscript from Athos (Ill. 02 page 51). Here we see Cosmas and Damian standing round the bed. It is the portrayal of a cure. Some other (posthumous) miracles are portrayed too. A similar image is to be found in the museum of the Chiesa di San Giorgio dei Greci in Venice (Ill. 48 page 111). It was painted around 1600 by Tzanfournaris. Although he too is a Greek painter, he worked and lived in Venice at the time and must have been familiar with the legend of the transplant of the black leg. In this icon as well other miracles are portrayed apart from the miracle of the black leg. In his book on Cosmas and Damian in Italy Maggioni writes that one of the miracles in this icon is indeed about the miracle of the transplant.

It is remarkable that in the last few years I have managed to add many Spanish illustrations to my collection. It appeared there were many of them whose existence I did not know of. In my search for these 'lacking' Spanish illustrations I made the acquaintance of art historian Carmen Fracchia. She considers the illustrations of the miracle of the black leg from a surprisingly different angle. She distinguishes clearly between the Spanish and other European illustrations. This distinction is quite clear in the chapter that she has contributed to this book. Furthermore I received illustrations from countries outside Europe: the USA, Mexico and Brazil. My friend Dimitros Kokkinakis from Chios (Greece) sent me a number of (modern) Greek illustrations originating from various churches and the Chios museum (Ill. 72, 78-81 pages 147, 153-156). The photograph of the picture of the miracle on an altar painted by Sebastián López Dávalos in Mexico City cathedral (Ill. 52 page 115) makes the series of illustrations in this book very special and exclusive. Up to now the only photograph of this picture available was in black and white in an article on the painter by Rogelio Ruiz Gomar. Owing to Dr. Dick Papousek's efforts and tenacity I obtained a color photograph to include in my book.

Sometimes one has to take quite a lot of pains to make the collection as complete as possible: in a Dutch book on saints the small town of Llo is mentioned, tucked away in the far Pyrenees. There is the description of a small chapel containing a polychrome wooden altar dedicated to Cosmas and Damian. On one of the panels the transplanting of the black leg is depicted. The journey to (La) Llo was wonderful, especially the final stage into the mountains. At first there was the feeling of excitement because the small town really existed: there was a small church, but no chapel. Then the big disappointment: in the small church no Cosmas and Damian, let alone an altar dedicated to them. So this was a dead end. Some years later Pierre Julien sent me an article about a Cosmas and Damian altar in La Llau. This must indicate the same altar as the one supposedly situated in (La) Llo. To be sure, in the Pyrenees not only the small town of La Llo but also La Llau is to be found. Again we set off to the French Pyrenees. We drove from Amélie les Bains via a winding country road up to La Llau. One house, one farm, one shed and, hidden behind some shrubbery, a small chapel, that was La Llau. The chapel was firmly locked and had no windows. Apart from a dog, hardly alert, the hamlet left a sleepy impression. There was no reply when we rang the doorbell of the house and the farm. Because it was siesta time we decided to wait for a few hours. Our waiting was rewarded when the farmer arrived. He managed to tell us that the small chapel belonged to a relative, Henri Sors, a pharmacist in Amélie les Bains. The house in La Llau was his summer cottage. We also discovered that Mr. Sors used to visit La Llau for the weekends. We were assured that he would arrive that day, because he had not been seen the day before, Saturday. After an hour of waiting in vain we decided to return to Amélie les Bains. But Mr. Sors was not in his house in Amélie les Bains either. Might the farmer be right all the same? There was a fair chance that meanwhile Mr. Sors was at his summer cottage and it still being the weekend that he would probably have more time for us that day than the next one, a Monday, when his professional engagements might not enable him to come to La Llau. So we drove back into the mountains. And, to be sure, someone was working in the garden of the summer cottage and a 'city' car was parked in front of the door. We seemed to be in luck for Mr. Sors had indeed arrived. We explained who we were and what we wanted. We were given permission: of course we were allowed to see the chapel and of course we were permitted to take pictures of the altar. There was a problem, however, the key to the small chapel was missing. This meant just driving back to Amélie les Bains again, in vain by the way. Fortunately the farmer appeared to have a spare key as well, so that we were able to get inside. And there were the real altar plus the picture of the black leg (Ill. 58 page 121).

One day I received a note from Marie Louise David-Danel: *'Cher monsieur, je crois vous rendre service en vous signalant un oeuvre répresentant le miracle de la jambe noire et dont je n'avais pas connaissance jusque'ici.'* This determined the next holiday destination. This work of art appeared to be exhibited in Bolzano after a thorough restoration. However, a big problem arose. The floor where the work of art was exhibited was closed due to work on the lighting precisely in the week of our visit to the museum. After we had explained that we had driven over 700 miles especially to see this work of art, a number of attendants adopted a more helpful attitude. Another part of the bored seated bunch obviously showed less cooperation. Between the two parties a discussion arose that we did not fully comprehend. Some of them clearly wanted to do us a favour by making an exception. The other party did not want to move an inch, for certain reasons that we were to understand later. To overcome the deadlock we wished to see the managing director, but the reaction was negative. As it happened he was in a meeting owing to a staff crisis. This was no surprise to us and it explained the somewhat peculiar attitude of the attendants. After a lot of pleading one of the cooperative attendants finally fetched the managing director for us. From that moment there were no further problems. The locked museum wing was opened especially for us, the lights were lit and the plastic cloths were removed from the works of art. We were given permission to photograph what we wanted, which we did of course. Slightly embarrassed, because we thought that the staff crisis had reached a climax by our doing, we left the museum (Ill. 20 page 69).

Pierre Julien (‘*selon nous*’) had informed me that a picture of the miracle might be portrayed on the altar of the Church of Cosmas and Damian in Hontoria del Pinar in Spain. During one of our recent holidays we called at Hontorio del Pinar where we soon found the church. On the edge of the small town is a graceful simple old church with a funny portico in which one finds two beardy worldly-looking saints: Cosmas and Damian. The church was locked, we had to search someone who could help us out. A man who was making a telephone call outside in the street was one of the few people we met in the almost deserted small town. I asked him when the church would open. He put his cell phone in my hand informing me that his girlfriend could help me out, for she spoke English, he didn’t. She told me she would inquire into when the church would be open. After some time the man returned with his cell phone. Again I spoke to his girlfriend. She had made inquiries and she was adamant that mass would be celebrated in the church at 8 p.m. the following day. Although our next holiday cottage was some 180 miles further on, we decided to go there first and to return for the black leg the following day. Hontorio del Pinar did not have a hotel and, moreover, we did not want to run the risk that our cottage would be assigned to others if we did not arrive in time. We knew what we were in for, and we were determined to face the long drives. The following day we drove back to Hontorio del Pinar through a landscape of impressive beauty. We were back at the church in good time. While waiting in front of the church our uncertainty increased: would there really be a mass at 8 o’clock and would there really be a picture of the miracle on the altar of this church and, if it were there, would it be visible and easily photographed. Sure enough, at quarter to eight the parish priest left his presbytery and walked to the church door. Inside we made his acquaintance. He was greatly interested and lit the lights of the church and there we saw the 17th century altar with, among other things, the picture of the miracle of the black leg (Ill. 55 page 118).

Of a completely different nature was laying hands on a Brazilian comic book with the illustration of the miracle of the transplant of the black leg. It is a religious booklet in a series of saints’ lives. Through others I had heard that in this ‘coleção Série Sagrada’ there existed a booklet on the lives and miracles of Cosmas and Damian: ‘História de São Cosme e São Damião’. For many years I tried to get hold of this booklet. It is only to be found in an antiquarian bookshop. Ordering in Brazil repeatedly appeared unsuccessful, perhaps impossible. Also relatives of mine with connections in Brazil seemed to fail in having it sent to them. When I had almost given up, somebody from Brazil happened to respond to an e-mail request I had sent at least two years previously. After some e-mail correspondence and after having paid the booklet would be forwarded to me. Within a few days it was indeed delivered! A few months later, through my cousin Jessica Teunissen, I received a second copy which had unexpectedly been sent to her after all. In the booklet the life of Cosmas and Damian is recorded as Jacob de Voragine wrote it down in the *Legenda Aurea*. At the end the three posthumous miracles are depicted as well. The booklet is written like a comic book, completely according to the medieval tradition, but then in a 20th century version, including 'balloon texts'. To be true, it is not a work of art, but still so odd that this was reason enough to include this illustration of the miracle of the black leg in this book (Ill. 66 page 141).

Up to now there is only one picture I couldn't trace. Pierre Julien – who always sent me correct information - sent me the details about a picture. It is made by Fernando Lopez in the 17th century, it should be in the museum of the Diocese in Malaga. It depicts the wonder of the transplantation. The work is not exposed in the museum, the personnel in the museum is convinced it is in the depot, but all efforts to receive a photograph of it failed unfortunately.

In the book now before you more than 80 photos of works of art have been collected. A miniature from the *Legenda Aurea* in the Huntington Library in S. Marino, California, end 13th century (Ill. 01 page 50), is the earliest illustration of the miracle. This edition of the *Legenda Aurea* is extraordinary because of the splendid miniatures accompanying all of the saint's stories. The Huntington library also granted me permission to include the complete text of the saint's story of Cosmas and Damian in their manuscript of the *Legenda Aurea*. To do so, it was necessary for me to have at my disposal a photo of a page without illustrations (fol. 132v.) which was not yet available in their internet files. I owe it to the efforts made by the classicist Professor Ellen Finkelpearl, one of my wife's colleagues, that the Huntington Library had a photograph of that page in the *Legenda Aurea* made available to me (Ill. I,II pages 22, 23). For the translation of the chapter on the saints Cosmas and Damian from the *Legenda Aurea* I again chose William Granger Ryan's translation, revised according to the edition Maggioni.

The book contains four illustrations before 1400. 43 Paintings and sculptures were produced in the 15th and 16th century. Ten were made in the 17th century. After that, the miracle is less often depicted. I have only been able to find four that originate from between 1700 and 1900. After 1900 the subject seems to receive more attention in art. From 1900 to the present 20 illustrations have been collected. That the number of illustrations made of this miracle decreases quite drastically can for the greater part be explained by the then increasing skepticism towards extremely miraculous events such as the replacement of a leg. Urged by criticism from protestants and the outcome of the Council of Trent, held from 1545 to 1564, the Roman Catholic Church closely scrutinized the credibility of the saints and their numerous legends. Extraordinary miracles such as the transplant of a complete leg from then on were seen more as superstition than as a miracle. If we take a closer look at the illustrations after this period, what strikes us is the fact that in quite a number the character of the illustration changes (see also de Jong's chapter in this book). Before that time a miracle is depicted, from now more and more a surgical operation is represented. Instruments appear and sometimes blood. In some illustrations we see that the verger on the receiving end has to be contained owing to pain suffered during surgery. Cosmas and Damian are no longer the only ones involved in the miracle. On the illustrations after 1650 we more often see the Holy Virgin or angels being depicted who from a sky opening itself direct the surgery that is executed. Cosmas and Damian have turned into intermediaries who can only perform miracles thanks to higher powers.

All but seven of the illustrations have been found in Europe. Most of the five illustrations from the USA also originate from Europe. Divided up by country of origin (the country possessing the work of art at present) the distribution is as follows:

Spain	21
Italy	19
France	14
USA	5
Greece	6
United Kingdom	3
Germany	3
Switzerland	2

Austria, Belgium, Brazil, Malta, Mexico, the Netherlands and Portugal 1 each.

So the majority of illustrations of the miracle of the black leg is found in Spain, Italy and France. This is even more conspicuous if we mainly focus on illustrations earlier than the 19th century. To this may be added that they also include some 'stray' ones from outside Europe that originate from Italy and Spain. As a consequence classification according to country of origin or country where illustrations are shown nowadays does not make much sense. In this book I have arranged the illustrations more or less chronologically. I have divided them into three groups; the 'classic' ones (illustrations up to around 1500), the illustrations dating from the 16th up to and including the 19th century and the modern ones. These three groups of illustrations have been inserted in between the chapters.

Most of the sites where illustrations are to be found I visited myself. On almost all of the 'black leg missions' my wife Maaike was my companion. She did most of the talking while I managed to concentrate on the photography. This project would not have succeeded without her. Moreover, we were left with unforgettable holidays. Some of the many exciting searches have been described above.

Acknowledgements

I owe many thanks to my co-authors Carmen Fracchia, Catrien Santing and Jan de Jong. Without any hesitation they agreed to write a contribution for this new volume. In her chapter Carmen Fracchia sheds some light on the specific part played by the Spanish illustrations of the miracle. Catrien Santing offers an insideful investigation into the interrelation of religion and medicine in the Middle Ages. Jan de Jong has completely revised the earlier version in the preceding volume. Thanks to these authors the book now contains a number of very fascinating historical and art-historical chapters. I owe a debt of gratitude to Piet van Riel who corrected the English in some chapters.

Without the financial assistance of various institutions it would have been impossible to publish this book.

O.I.M. (Orthopedische Instrument Makerij) in Assen (the Netherlands) has enabled the publication of a second edition by their financial contribution.

I am grateful to the subdivision Transplantation and Organ Donation of the Department of Surgery of the UMCG (University Medical Centre Groningen, the Netherlands) for its contribution.

I also express my gratitude to the Chios Pharmacy Museum (Greece) for its financial support.

Due to Carmen Fracchia's efforts, the Ministerio de Ciencia e Innovación (Spain) has with a gift contributed to the full color reproductions.

When I told Roelf Barkhuis of my plan to publish a second version of 'One Leg in the Grave' he immediately enthusiastically showed his interest in publishing this volume. Thanks to Barkhuis Publishing it has turned into a splendid edition.

Literature

Avalon, J. 1923. 'La greffe humaine dans l'art', *Aesculape*, 8-10.

Boureau, A. 2004. *Jacques de Voragine, La Légende dorée*, Paris.

Cassar, P. 1972. 'The Cult and Iconography of Saints Cosmas and Damian in the Maltese Islands', *Melita Historica*, 6 I 25-49.

'Còleção Serie Sagrada'. 1954. *História de São Cosme e São Damião*, Rio de Janeiro, 27-28.

David-Danel, M.-L. 1958. *Iconographie des saints médecins Côme et Damien*, Lille.

Deubner, L. 1907. *Kosmas und Damian. Texte und Einleitung*, Berlin.

Devaux, G. 2002. 'Les saints Côme et Damien dans l'ex-libris: deux nouvelles réalisations', *Revue d'histoire de la pharmacie*, 50, 334, 2e trim. 316-19.

Gonzalez, R. J. 1973. *Iconografía de los Santos Cosme y Damian*, Barcelona.

Goosen, L. 2008. *Van Afra tot de Zevenslapers. Heiligen uit Oost en West. Hun leven, de legendevorming, de verering en hun aanwezigheid in de kunsten*, Nijmegen.

Hilhorst-Böink, C., Hilhorst T. forthcoming. *Jacobus de Voragine, Legenda Aurea. Vertaling, inleiding en annotatie.*

Hood, W. 1993. *Fra Angelico at S. Marco*, New Haven/London.

Huisman, F.G. 1990. 'Cosmas en Damianus in de Groninger Martinikerk. Een uiting van ontluikend medisch standsbesef?', *Groningse Volksalmanak*, 39-67.
Julien, P. 1993. 'Apport de l'iconographie des Saints Côme et Damien à l'histoire de la médecine et de la pharmacie', *Conférence de l'institut d'Histoire de la médecine,* 43-50.
Julien, P. 1973. 'La confrérie des saints Côme et Damien a Luzarches', *Revue d'Histoire de la Pharmacie* 21, 218.
Julien, P. 1997. 'Un tableau italien du XVIe siècle retrouvé', *Revue d'Histoire de la Pharmacie,* 314, 226.
Julien, P. 1998. 'Le miracle de la jambe noire dans l'art', *Revue d'Histoire de la Pharmacie,* 473-76.
Julien, P. 1968. 'Saint Côme et saint Damien en leur chapelle de La Llau (Pyrénées-Orientales)', *Histoire des sciences médicales,* 147-54.
Kaftal, G. 1952. *Iconography of the Saints in Tuscan Painting,* Florence.
Kokkinakis, D. 2011. 'Un'icona ortodossa del miracolo della gamba nera inedita del monastero Agàthonos a Fthiotida in Grecia', *Atti e memorie, Rivista di Storia della Farmacia,* 28, 18-28.
López Campuzano, J. 1988. 'Iconografía de los Santos Sanadores (II): San Cosme y San Damián', *Anales de Historia del Arte,* 255-66.
Maggioni, F. 2011, *Ricerche Iconografia dei Santi Cosma e Damiano,* Conselve (It.).
Maggioni, F., Maggioni G., Talmelli D. 2005. *Santi Cosma e Damiano in Italia,* Conselve (It.).
Maggioni, F., Talmelli D., Maggioni G. 2009. *Anatomia di un Miracolo,* Conselve (It.).
Maggioni, G.P., Stella, F. 2007. *Iacopo da Varazze, Legenda Aurea* (Edizione Nazionale dei Testi Mediolatini 20), Florence.
Peyrí i Rocamora, J. 1932. *Iconografia d'uns Metges Anargirs: Sant Cosme I Sant Damià*, Barcelona.
Ruiz Gomar, R. 1993. 'Sebastián López Dávalos, un pintor novohispano del siglo XVII', *Anales del Instituto de Investigaciones estéticas,* 16, 64, 15-29.
Ryan, W.G. 1993. *Jacobus de Voragine. The golden legend* vol. 2, Princetown.
Shapley, F.R. 1966-1973. *Paintings from the Samuel H. Kress collection,* Washington.
Zimmerman, K.W. (ed.). 1998. *One Leg in the Grave,* Maarssen (NL).

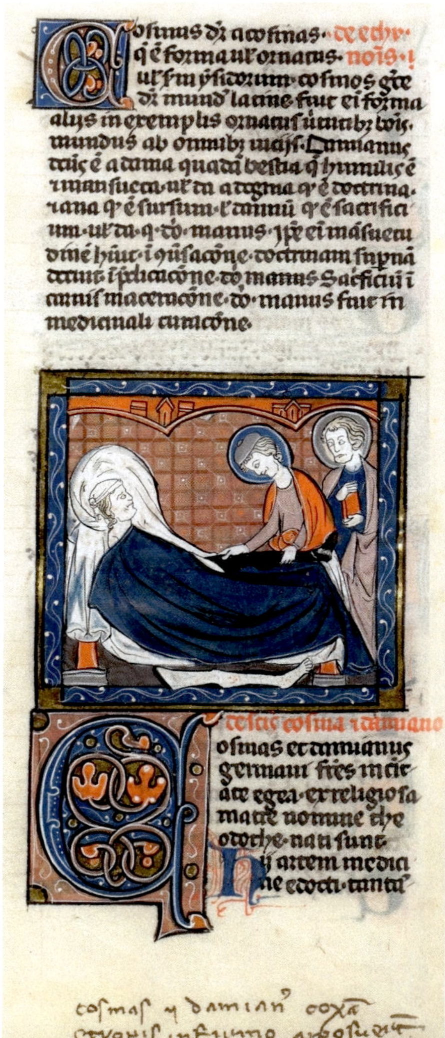

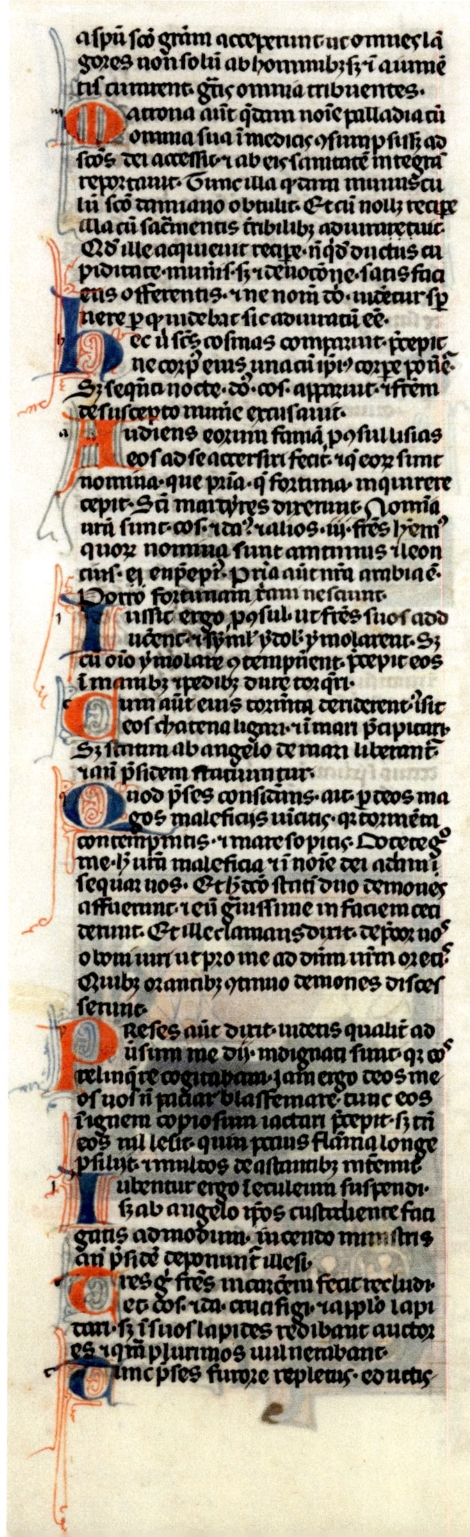

I. **Anonymous,** *Legenda Aurea* HM 3027 fol. 132r, 132v, late 13th century. Henry E. Huntington Library, San Marino (U.S.A.).

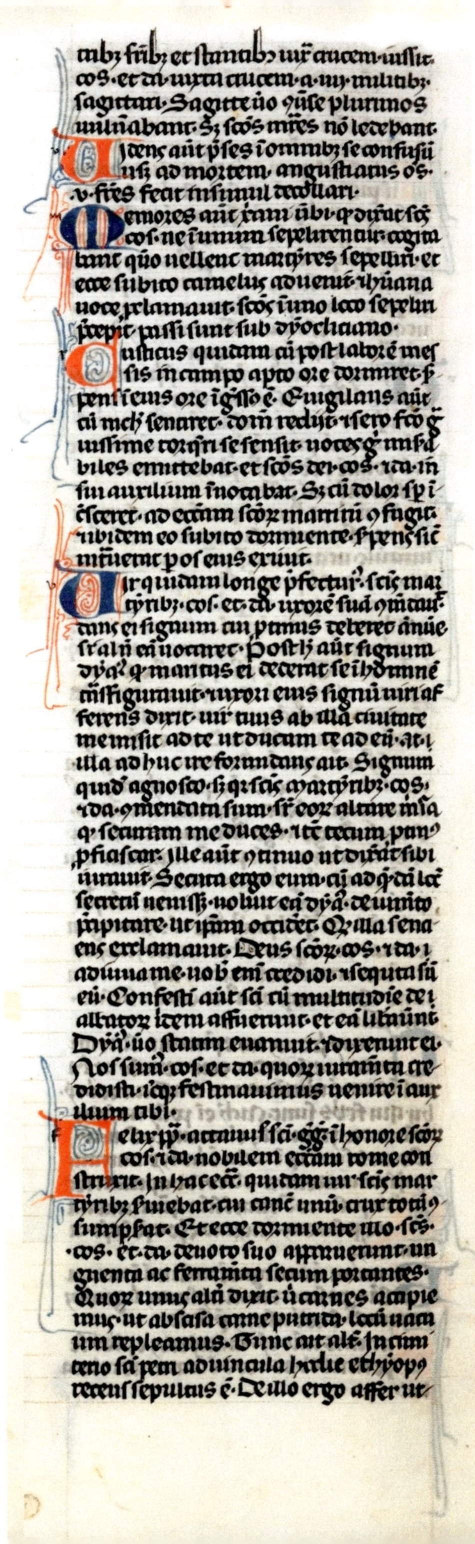

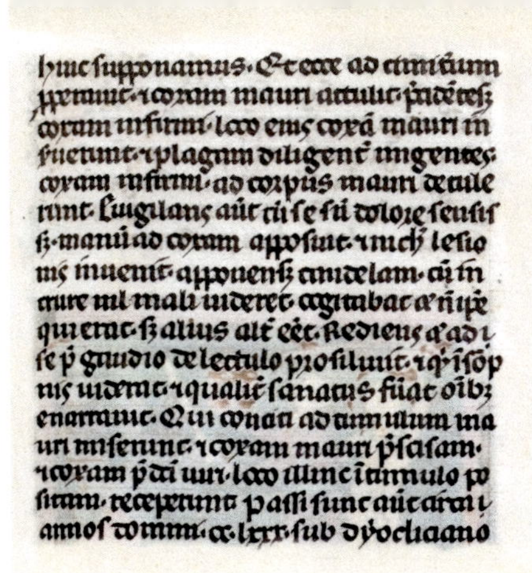

II. **Anonymous,** *Legenda Aurea* HM 3027 fol.132v, 133r, late 13th century. Henry E. Huntington Library, San Marino (U.S.A.).

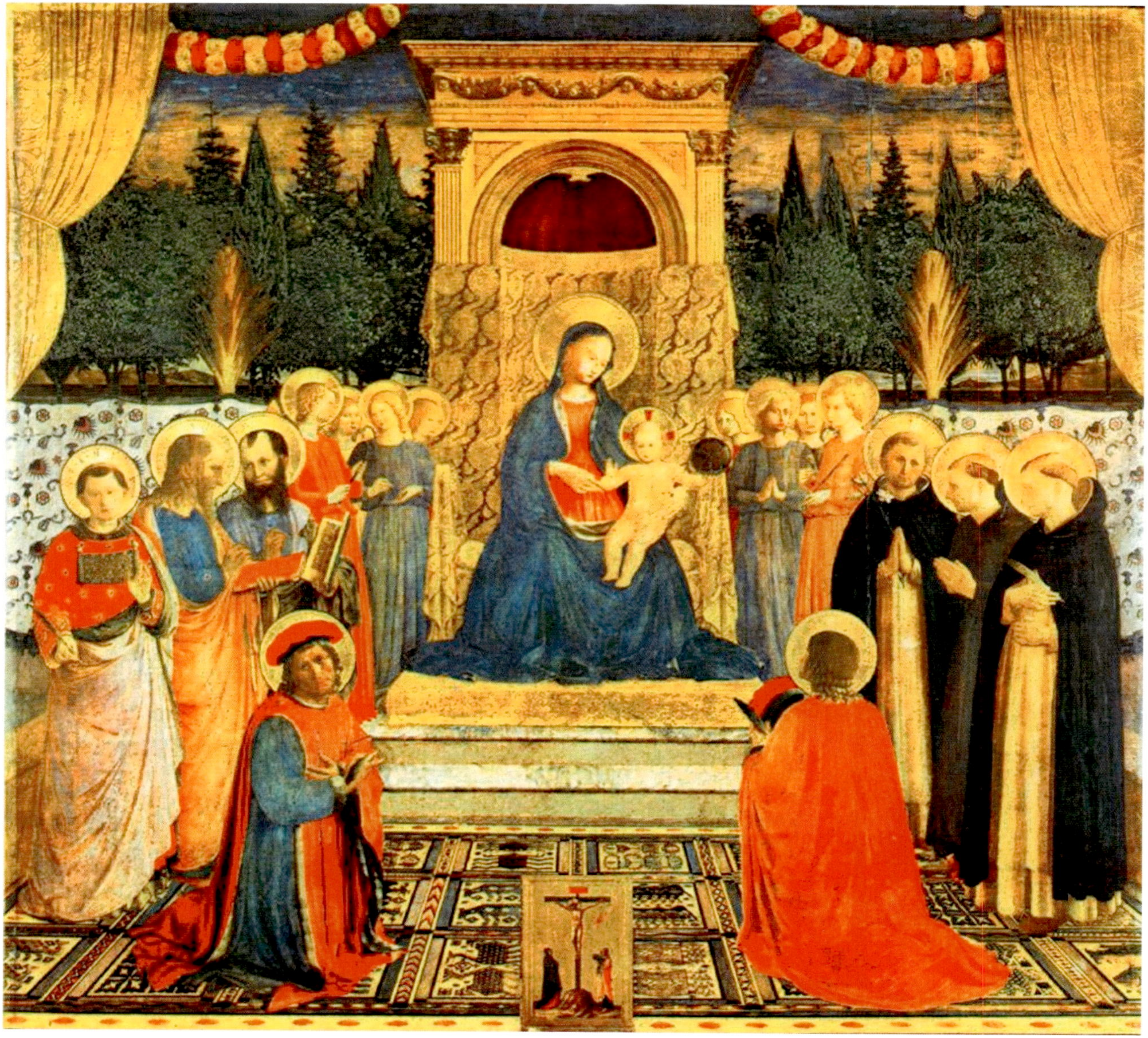

III. **Fra Angelico** (ca. 1387–1455), *main panel altarpiece*, 1442. Museo di S. Marco, Florence (Italy).

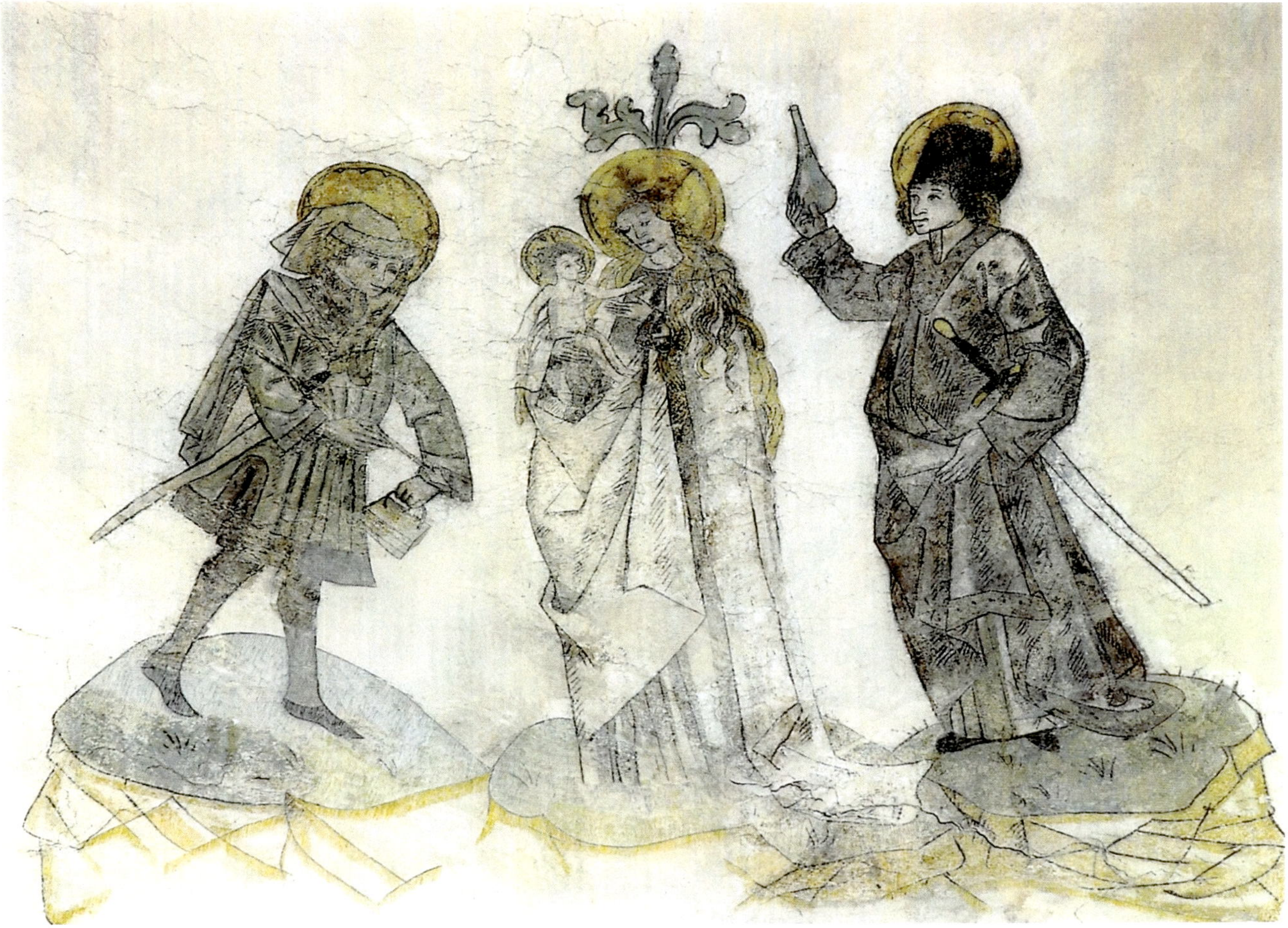

IV. **Anonymous,** *fresco,* 1482-1490. Martinikerk, Groningen (the Netherlands).

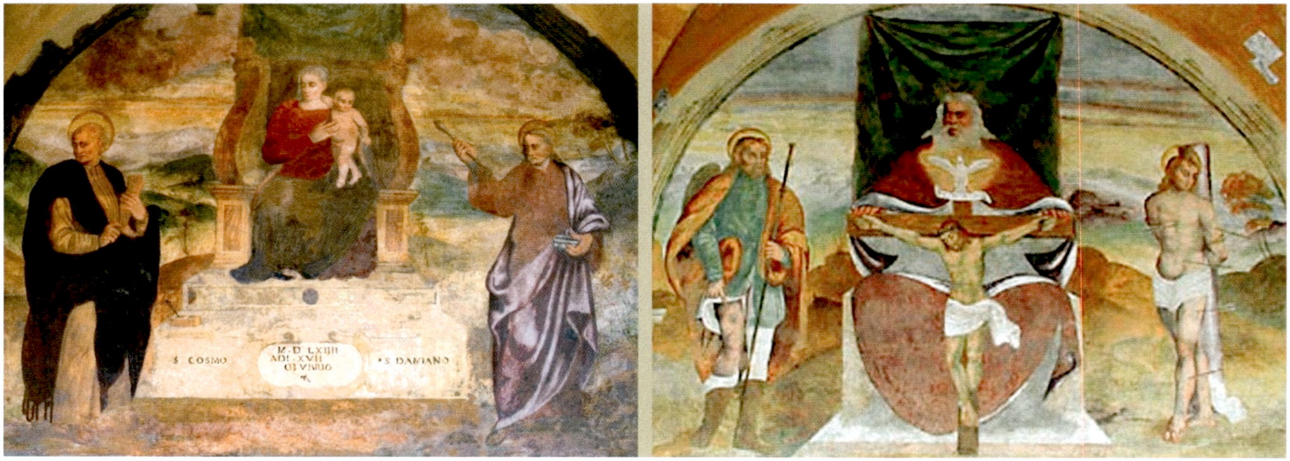

V. **Antonio da Tisoi (**ca.1485-1564), *fresco,* left and right sides of the entrance porch, 1564. S. Rocco, Belluno (Italy).

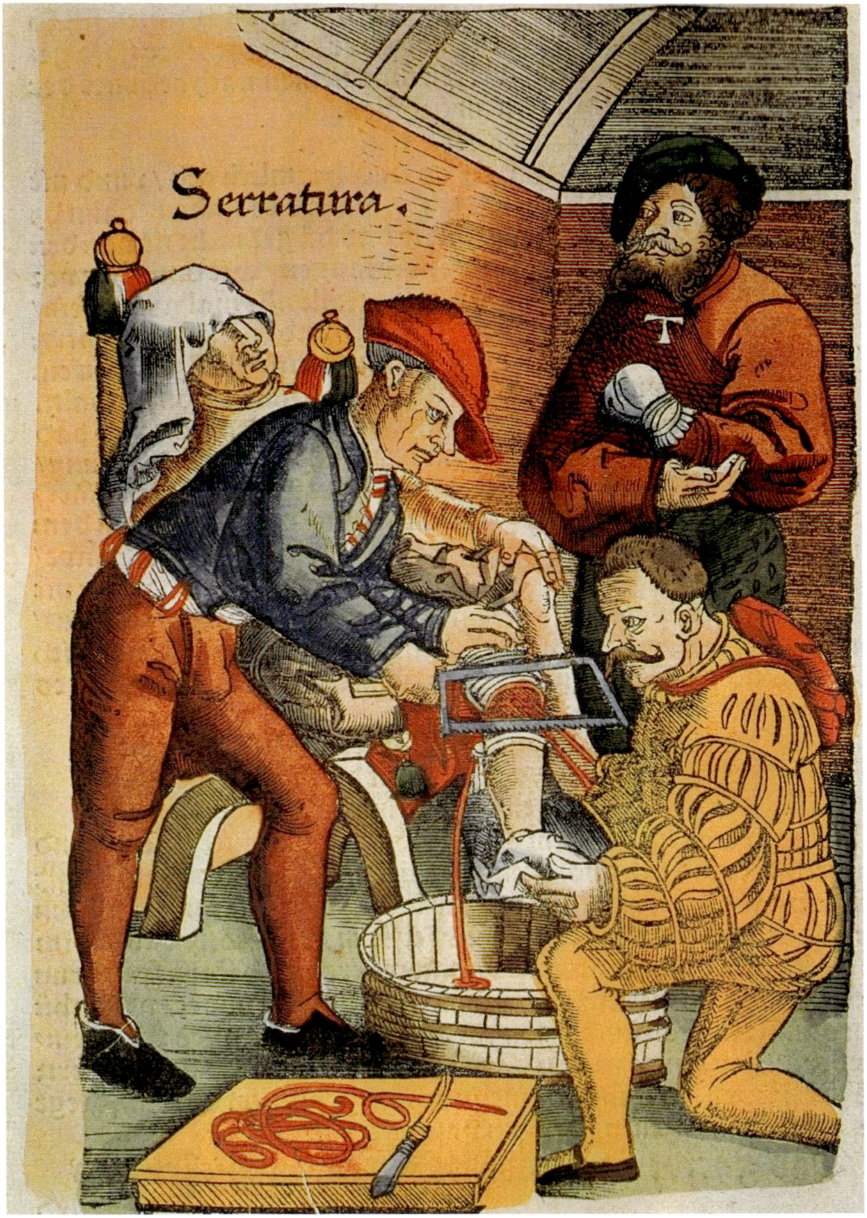

VI. **Hans von Gersdorff,** *Feldtbuch der Wundartzney* (Strasbourg, 1517).

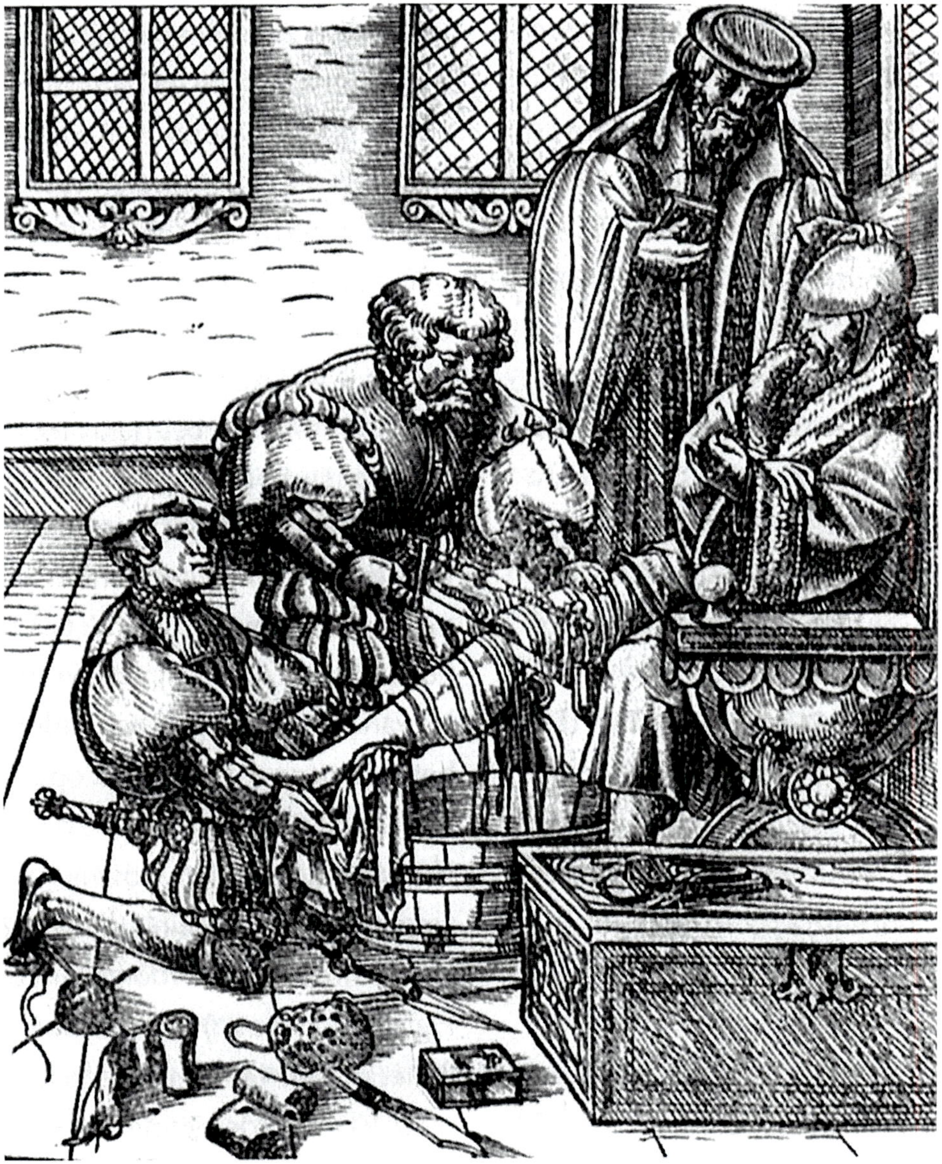

VII. **Walther Hermann Ryff,** *Die grosse Chirurgei* (Frankfurt a. M., 1545).

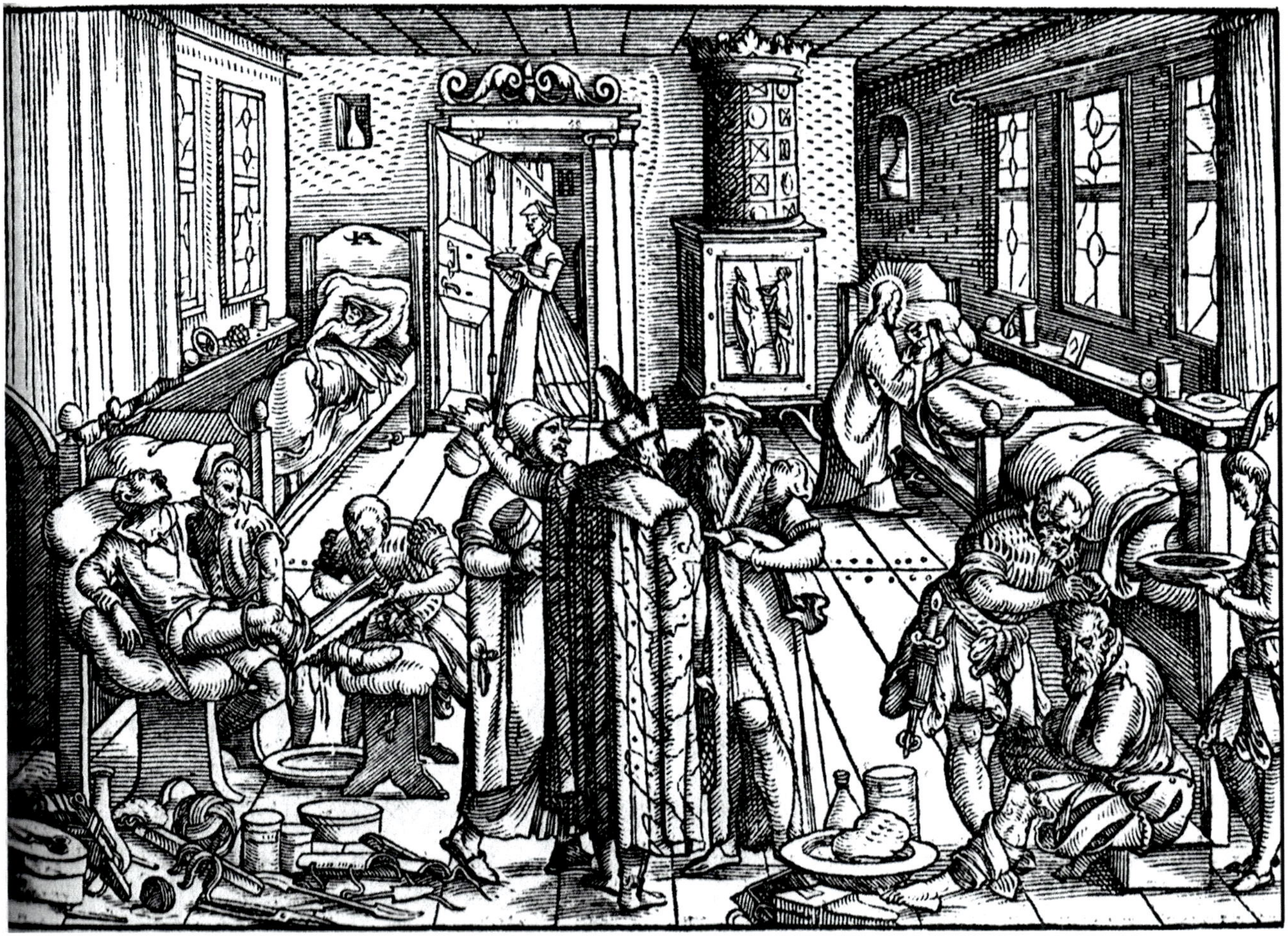

VIII. **Theophrastus Paracelsus,** *Opus Chyrurgicum.... Wund und Artzneybuch* (Frankfurt a.M., 1566).

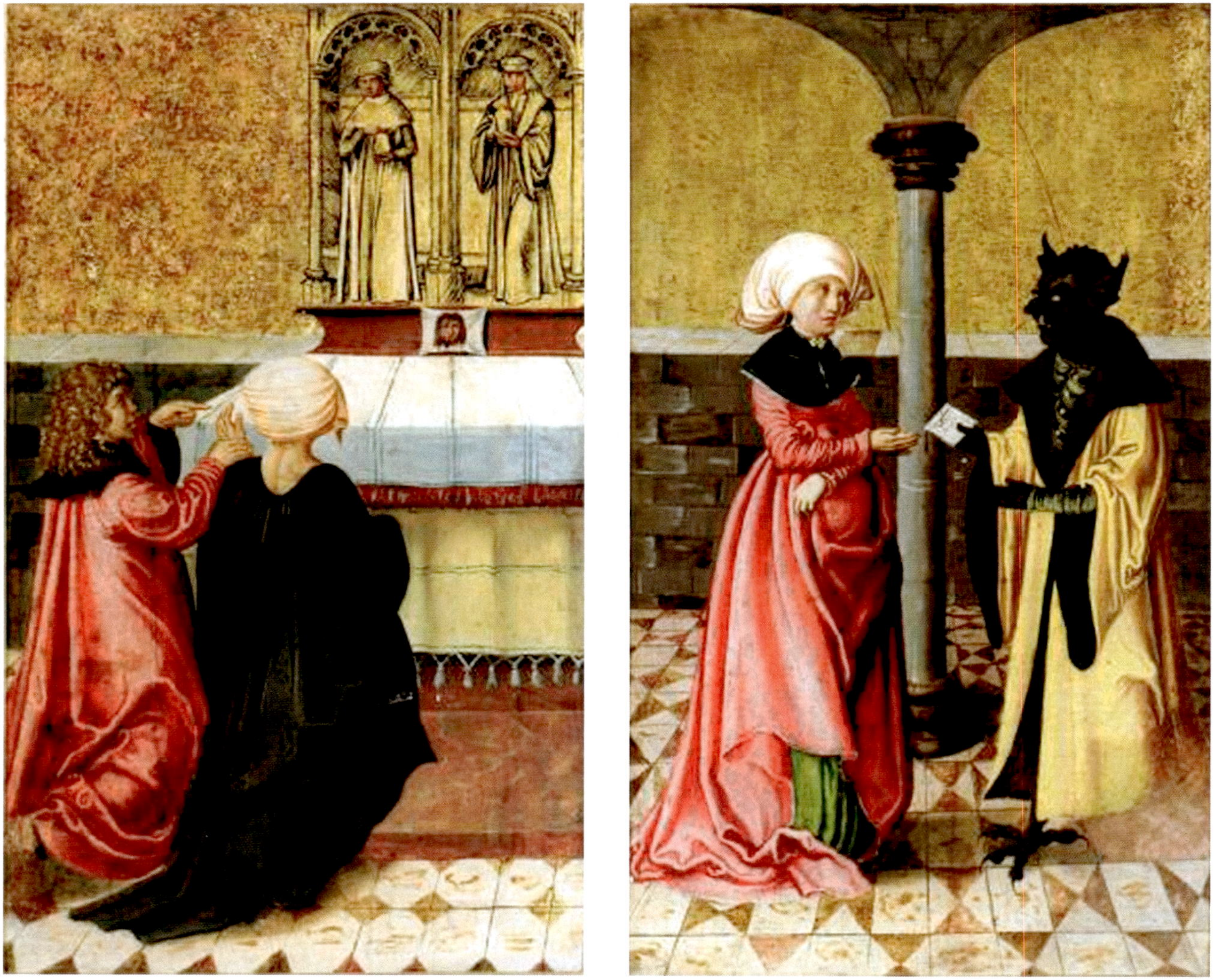

IX. **"Master of the Legend Scenes",** *panels transferred to canvas,* early 16th century. Österreichische Galerie Belvedere, Vienna (Austria).

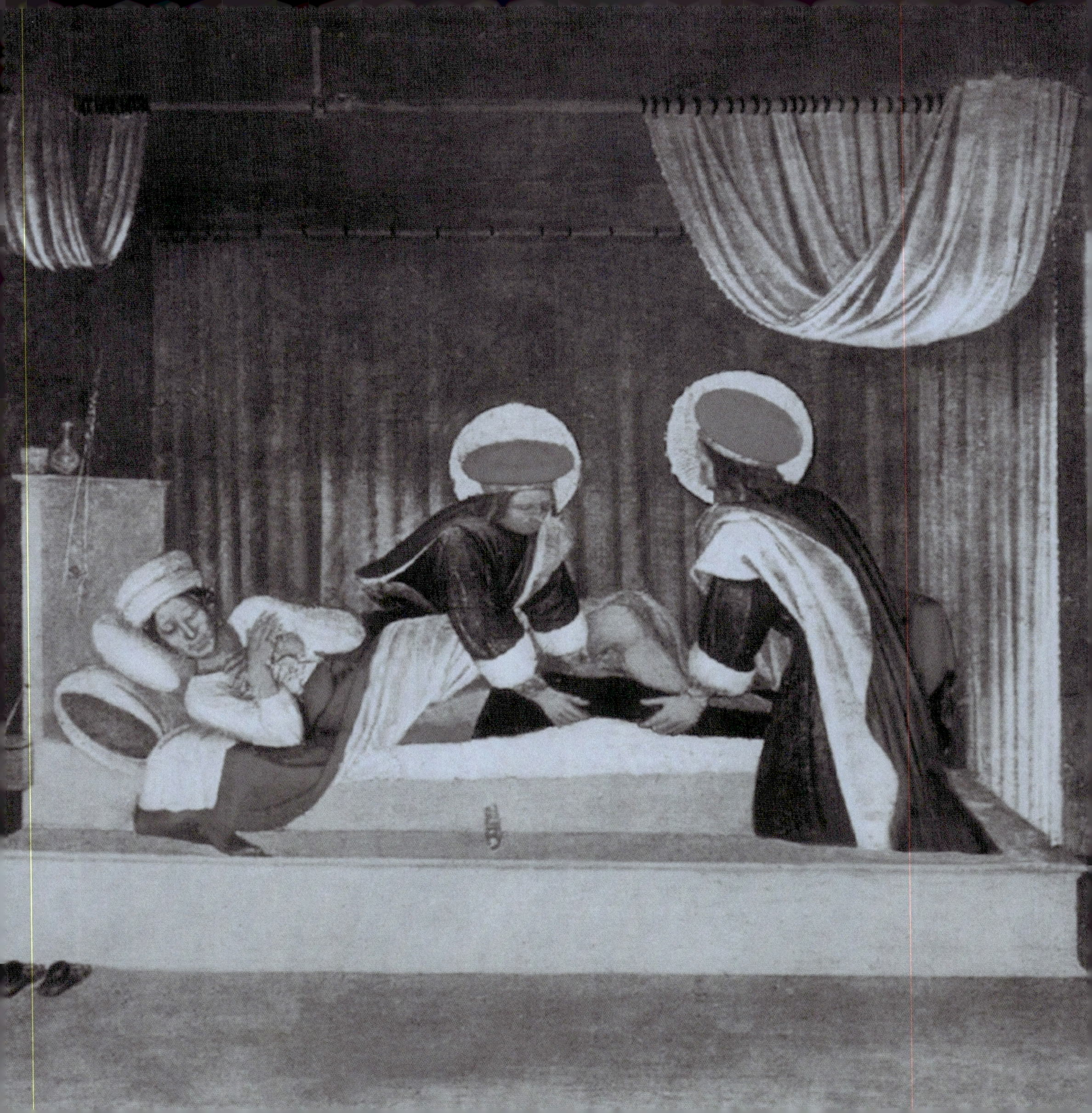

Jacobus de Voragine, the Golden Legend: saints Cosmas and Damian

(edition G.P.Maggioni, Firenze-Milano 2007, page 1094-1099)

Translated by William Granger Ryan *(revised according to the edition by G.P. Maggioni)*

The name Cosmas comes from *cosmos*, which means form or adorned. Or, according to Isidore, *cosmos* is the Greek word for clean, as is the Latin word *mundus*. Saint Cosmas was a form, an example to others; he was adorned with good virtues and clean of all vices. Damianus, or Damian, is derived from *dama*, a humble, gentle beast, or the name comes from *dogma*, doctrine, and *ana*, above, or from *damium*, which is sacrifice. Or Damianus is equivalent to *Domini manus*, the hand of the Lord. Saint Damian was mild of manner, had supernal doctrine in his preaching, was a sacrifice in the mortification of his flesh, and was the hand of the Lord in the healing cures he brought about.

Cosmas and Damian were brothers, born of a pious mother, Theodora by name, in the city of Egea. They learned the art of medicine from the Holy Spirit and received such grace from the Holy Spirit that they cured the illnesses not only of men and women but of animals, not taking any payment for their services. A lady named Palladia, however, who had spent all she had on doctors, came to the saints of God and by them was fully restored to health. She therefore secretly offered a gift to Saint Damian and, when he declined to accept it, appealed to him with solemn oaths. He then accepted the gift, not that he was greedy for the money but to satisfy the donor's kind intention, as well as to avoid seeming to dishonor the name of the Lord, since the woman had adjured him in that name. When Saint Cosmas learned of this, he gave orders that his body was not to be buried with his brother's, but the following night the Lord appeared to Cosmas and explained Damian's reason for his action.

Word of the brothers' fame reached Lisias, the proconsul, and he had them summoned and asked them their names, their native land, and their possessions. The holy martyrs replied: 'Our names are Cosmas and Damian; we have three brothers named Antimus, Leontius, and Euprepius; Arabia is our homeland; and as for earthly fortunes, Christians do not acquire them.' The proconsul ordered them to fetch their brothers, and then to sacrifice to the idols together. When the five brothers unanimously refused to sacrifice, Lisias commanded that they be tortured in their hands and feet. They made light of these torments, and he ordered them to be bound with chains and thrown into the sea, but at once they were drawn out by an angel and set before the judge. This official gave thought to the matter and said: 'By the great gods, it is by sorcery that you conquer, because you mock at torments and calm the sea! Therefore teach me your magic arts, and in the name of the god Adrian I will follow you.' No sooner had he said this than two demons appeared and struck him in the face with great force, and he cried out: 'I beg you, good men, to pray for me to your God!' They prayed, and the demons disappeared. The judge said: 'You see how angry the gods are with me because I thought of leaving them. Now therefore I will not suffer you to blaspheme my gods!' He ordered them to be thrown into a huge fire, but the flame not only left the martyrs unharmed, but leapt out and slew many bystanders. The brothers were then stretched on the rack, but an angel kept them uninjured, and the torturers, tired of beating them, returned them to the judge. He in turn had three of the brothers put back in prison, but ordered Cosmas and Damian to be crucified and stoned by the crowd. The stones turned back upon the throwers and wounded a great number. The judge, now beside himself with rage, had the three brothers brought out and ranged around the cross, while four soldiers shot arrows at Cosmas and Damian, still crucified; but the arrows turned and struck many, while the holy martyrs remained untouched. The judge, defeated at every turn, was at death's door from frustration and had the five brothers beheaded together. The Christians, remembering what Saint Cosmas had said about not burying him with Damian, wondered how and where the holy martyrs wanted to be buried, when suddenly a camel appeared on the scene, spoke in a human voice, and ordered the saints to be entombed in one place. They suffered under Diocletian, who began to reign about A.D. 287.

A peasant, after hours of working at the harvest, fell asleep in the field with his mouth open, and a snake slipped into his mouth and down to his belly. The man woke up and felt nothing, and went on home, but by evening suffered severe pains in the stomach. He uttered pitiful cries and invoked the aid of Cosmas and Damian, saints of God, but the pain grew worse and he ran to the church of the holy martyrs. There he suddenly fell asleep, and the snake slipped out of his mouth as it had slipped in.

A man who was about to set out on a long journey commended his wife to the care of the holy martyrs Cosmas and Damian, and gave her a sign that she could rely on if at any time he called her. Afterwards the devil, knowing the sign the husband had given, got himself up as a man, showed the woman the sign, and said: 'Your husband sent me to you from that city to conduct you to him.' She was afraid to go, and said: 'I recognize the sign, but I am commended to the holy martyrs Cosmas and Damian, so you must swear to me on their altar that you will take me safely to him.' The devil immediately swore as requested. The woman went with him, and when they came to a secluded spot, the devil wanted to throw her off her horse and kill her. When she felt danger coming, she exclaimed: 'O God of saints Cosmas and Damian, help me! I trusted both of you and followed this man!' Instantly the saints appeared with a host of men clad in white and set the woman free. The devil vanished. They said to her: 'We are Cosmas and Damian, in whose oath you trusted and we hurried to come to your assistance.'

Pope Felix, a predecessor of Saint Gregory, built a noble church in Rome in honor of Saints Cosmas and Damian. In this church there was a man, a devoted servant of the holy martyrs. One of the man's legs was already totally consumed by a cancer. While he was asleep, the two saints appeared to their devoted servant, bringing salves and surgical instruments. One of them said to the other: 'Where can we get flesh to fill in where we cut away the rotted leg?' The other said: 'Just today an Ethiopian was buried in the cemetery of Saint Peter in Chains. Go and take his leg and we'll put it in place of the bad one.' So he sped to the cemetery and brought back the Moor's leg, and the two saints cut off the sick man's leg and inserted the Moor's in its place, carefully anointing the wound. Finally they took the amputated leg and attached it to the body of the dead Moor. The man woke up, felt no pain, put his hand to his leg, and detected no lesion. He held a candle to the leg and could see nothing wrong with it, and began to wonder whether he was himself or somebody else. Then he came to his senses, bounded joyfully from his bed, and told everyone about what he had seen in his dreams and how he had been healed. They sent at once to the Moor's tomb, and found that his leg had indeed been cut off and the aforesaid man's limb put in its place in the tomb.

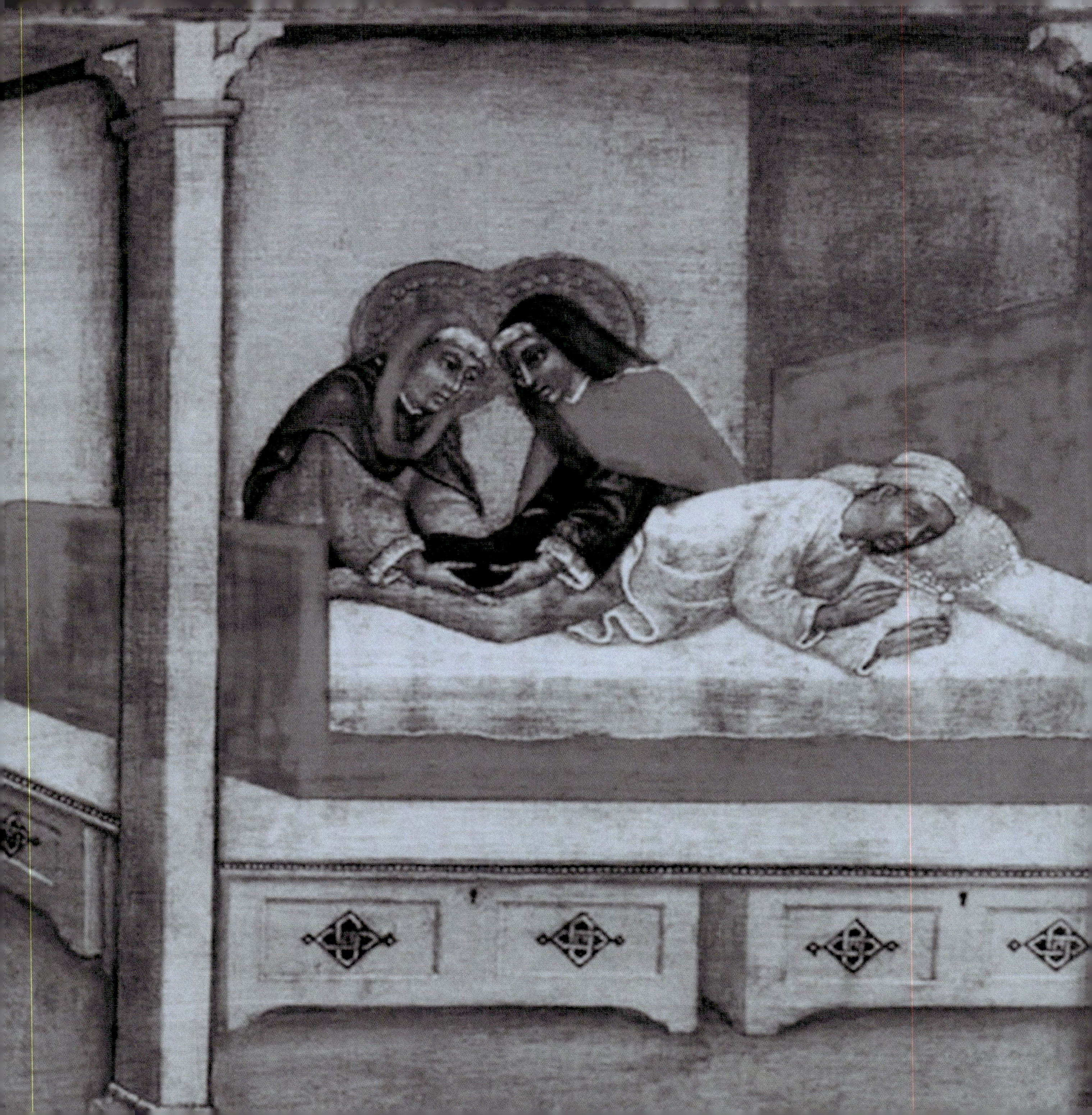

Transplantation and salvation

Jan L. de Jong

Like most other legends, the Miracle of the Black Leg is not an account of a fact, but a story to inspire awe, reverence and devotion. In the version of *The Golden Legend*, Cosmas and Damian are portrayed as faithful devotees of Christ, carrying out the exhortations to his followers. In *Mark* 6 (7-14), Christ had sent forth his disciples two by two and charged them to take nothing for their journey: 'no bread, no wallet, no money'. In addition, he had charged them to preach that men should repent, to cast out devils and to heal the sick. Cosmas and Damian met these demands perfectly. What is more, the healing of the leg consumed by cancer not only fulfils the charge to heal the sick, but corresponds in its structure closely to the prototype of other miracle stories and biblical accounts of wondrous healings. The pattern of these tales consists of a person who is incurably ill or injured; (s)he is healed by Christ or a saint; the cured person is highly amazed and grateful to God; the people who have witnessed the miraculous healing also express their admiration and are either confirmed in their Christian faith or convert to it.

Just like the legend itself, pictures showing the Miracle of the Black Leg were not meant to represent a factual truth either. They were made to represent the story visually for those who could not read, and inspire them to reverence and devotion. These pictures should therefore not be seen as documents of surgical practice of their time, even though the persons in them, as well as their surroundings, have usually been represented in contemporary terms. This, however, was general practice, meant to adapt the story to the world and the lives of the observers, so that they could relate to it more easily. This appears, for example, from a passage in an Italian handbook on prayer for young girls, written in 1454 and called *Zardino de Oration* (*Garden of Prayer*). Using the example of Christ's passion, it exhorts the readers to consider the story in the following way:

> The better to impress the story of the Passion on your mind, and to memorize each action of it more easily, it is helpful and necessary to fix the places and people in your mind: a city, for example, which will be the city of Jerusalem – taking for this purpose a city that is well known to you. In this city, find the principal places in which all the episodes of the Passion would have taken place [...] And then too you must shape in your mind some people, people well-known to you, to represent for you the people involved in the Passion...

Local Traditions and Variations

Legends like the Miracle of the Black Leg were spread over large parts of the Christian world and landed in widely divergent cultures. In each region and every time period, they may have meant something different, depending on the diverse backgrounds and particular local customs of the various societies. In Spain, for example, black people were more common than in other parts of Europe. They usually had a low social status and often were slaves. Thus, the story of a 'superior' white man whose leg was supplanted with that of a black person would mean something different from what it would in other societies, which were not or barely familiar with dark people, as we can read in the contribution by Carmen Fracchia.

In a time when written communication was relatively rare and the exchange of stories and ideas would mainly happen orally, it was no wonder that legends developed all kinds of local variations and grew into various versions. 'Regularization' and 'standardization' were introduced only gradually. It was not until 1171 that the prerogative to declare a deceased person to be a saint was reserved to the pope, and it took another four centuries (1588) to establish the present procedure of canonization. The critical study of hagiographical texts ('lives of the saints') on a consistent scholarly basis started only in 1643, when the first volume of the *Acta Sanctorum* was published. From then on, these *Acts of the Saints* have generally been recognized as the official biographies of the saints of the Catholic Church. However, before this process of 'regularization' and 'standardization' began, there already existed a range of versions and variations of legends about Cosmas and Damian, which has had its impact on later centuries up to the present day. Thus, there are three pairs of Cosmas and Damian: those of Cilicia in Arabia, who are venerated in the Eastern Orthodox Church on October 17; those of Asia Minor or Mesopotamia, also venerated in the Orthodox Church, on November 1; and those who were martyred outside Rome and are venerated in the Roman Catholic Church, on September 26. (Originally, they were venerated on September 27, but in 1969 their feast was moved to the 26th, so that it would not be overshadowed by the feast of the (now) more popular St. Vincent de Paul. The Orthodox Church venerates the 'Roman' Cosmas and Damian on July 1.) That these distinctions were in practice not always as clear cut as they are described here, appears from a painting ascribed to Antonio da Tisoi in Belluno, north of Venice in Italy (Ill. 39 page 102). The painting in fresco is situated in the *portico* of the church of S. Rocco (St. Roch), to the left of the entrance porch. It shows both saints flanking the Madonna, who is sitting on a throne with the Christ child on her lap. St. Damian is standing on her left side, while St. Cosmas, on her right, is holding a black leg, obviously referring to the legend of the miraculous surgery. (Due to the painting's dirty condition, it is not immediately clear that the leg is indeed darkly colored.) On the throne of the Madonna is written an inscription: M.D.LXIIII ADI XVII OTVBRIO, meaning: '1564, on the seventeenth day of October'. This date refers to the day on which Cosmas and Damian are venerated in the Orthodox Church and would imply that the two saints represented here are those from Cilicia in Armenia, and not the martyrs adored in the Roman Catholic Church.

This is not implausible, as there had traditionally been strong contacts between Armenia and the Venetian region to which Belluno belonged. In fact, the oldest church of Belluno is dedicated to the holy Blaise (Blasius) from Armenia, a healing saint (just like Cosmas and Damian), who had died in the fourth century. Thus, it may be not surprising that Antonio da Tisoi's painting seems to refer to the Orthodox instead of the Roman Catholic saints Cosmas and Damian. At the same time, however, the influence of the Roman Catholic Church is also in sight, as appears from one specific detail in the painting: the black leg held by St. Cosmas. The story of the miraculous healing does not occur in the earliest legends about St. Cosmas and Damian. It is told in a number of Greek texts on the lives of the saints from later centuries, but none of them mentions the peculiar detail that Jacobus de Voragine was the first to relate in his *Golden Legend* from around 1255-1266, namely that the substituting leg was black. Consequently, representations of the Miracle of the Black Leg do not occur in the art of the Orthodox Church, while they can hardly have appeared in the Roman Catholic world before c. 1270. The earliest known representation of the Miracle dates, in fact, from around 1300 (Ill.01 page 50). The black leg held by St. Cosmas in Antonio da Tisoi's painting illustrates, together with the date of October 17, how various traditions in the veneration of Sts Cosmas and Damian came together in places such as Belluno, in the border region between the East and the West.

Places and Purposes

Many pictures of Cosmas and Damian served a more specific purpose on top of the general function of inspiring the viewers to reverence and devotion. There usually was a particular reason to represent just them and not some other saint. Their presence in a certain church or on a specific spot can often be explained by special circumstances. Thus, there was an immediate cause why Antonio da Tisoi was commissioned to represent Cosmas and Damian in Belluno. What exactly this was, can be understood with the help of a matching painting, made by the same artist on the other side of the entrance porch of the same church of S. Rocco (Ill. V page 26). It shows a similar composition, with the Holy Trinity (instead of St Mary and the Christ child) enthroned in the centre, flanked by the holy Roch and Sebastian, both saints who were especially invoked against the plague. An inscription added in the nineteenth century, that is undoubtedly repeating information from a former version, states that the church was built in 1561, out of gratitude to St Roch for releasing the city from the pest in 1530.[1] This easily explains the presence of Sts Roch and Sebastian in the painting on the right side of the entrance porch, and also makes it clear why the healing saints Cosmas and Damian were included in the matching painting on the left.

---

1 'Divo Rocho / ob pestem anno MDXXX fugatam / voto civium anno MDLXI exstructum / a fisco anno MDCCCVI sibi attributum / in profanos usus anno MDCCCXVII conversum / a nobile matrona anno MDCCCLVI redemptum / orphanis in adnexas aedes collectis traditum / et in nitorem pristinum restitutum / Divo Rocho / domenica prima octobris anno MDCCCLX / iterum dedicatum'

Unfortunately, it is not always possible to trace the specific reason(s) for which a representation of Cosmas and Damian was made, apart from the general function. Unlike Antonio da Tisoi's paintings in Belluno, many pictures are no longer on the place they were initially made for. This makes it often hard to reconstruct their original context and, along with it, to find the particular reason why they came into being. In some cases, however, there seems to be enough information to make a good guess. Thus, the presence in Bremen of a sandstone relief from around 1400 (Ill. 07 page 56) could be explained by the fact that in 1334 the local Archbishop, Burchard Grelle, 'miraculously' retrieved relics of Cosmas and Damian, which had allegedly been immured in the choir of the cathedral. Archbishop Grelle claimed that they were the saints' skulls that his one-time predecessor Adaldag had brought from Rome, in 965. In an attempt to prevent that they would be forgotten again, Grelle had them transferred to a more dignified place in the Bremen cathedral, during a solemn Pentecost ceremony in 1335. Around 1420, they were put in a valuable shrine made of carved oak wood and covered with silver. Even though the exact details may need further clarification, it seems plausible that the origin of the sandstone relief from around 1400 should be seen in connection with the presence in Bremen of the relics of Cosmas and Damian, and with their special veneration in that city around that time.

Other than the relief, the shrine is no longer in Bremen. In 1649, when the city had become Lutheran, it was sold to Bishop Franz-Wilhelm von Wartenberg of Osnabrück, who passed it on to Elector Maximilian I of Bavaria. He had the shrine placed in St Michael's church in Munich, where it can still be seen. The skulls, however, remained in Bremen. Several centuries later, in 1964, Provost August Sandtel declared them 'probably not authentic', and in 1994 they were finally buried in the crypt of the local church of St Johann. The shrine, meanwhile, was put to a very appropriate use: it became the receptacle of another pair of skulls that were also claimed to be relics of Cosmas and Damian, and that are still kept in it. This makes the decorations inside the shrine hard to see. Among them are paintings by an unknown artist, showing the miracle of the black leg in two episodes (Ill. 08 page 57).

Particular circumstances may also explain how the picture in Vienna came into existence, although there is even less evidence than in the case of the Bremen relief. The painting (originally on panel, but transferred to canvas) dates from around 1500 and was made by an unknown artist, who is usually designated as 'the Master of the Legend Scenes' (Ill. 44 page 107). It probably formed part of a set or series of pictures, to which two paintings of similar height and related subjects belonged as well (also transferred to canvas and now in the Österreichische Galerie Belvedere in Vienna, Ill. IX page 30). They show, in two episodes, the legend of the wife saved from the devil by Cosmas and Damian. The provenance of the paintings does not go further back than the early twentieth century, when they were in the depot of the Kaiserliche Gemäldegalerie in Vienna. Perhaps they have always been in that city and were part of an altarpiece or another type of art work created for St. Stephen's Cathedral (Stephansdom). That church also claimed to possess the skulls of Cosmas and Damian! In 1413, a medical doctor commissioned a shrine for these relics, and in 1430 the members of the Medical Faculty made Cosmas and Damian their patron saints. Until far into the eighteenth century, the Faculty continued the tradition of yearly celebrating their feast. Possibly the paintings in Vienna should be seen in relation to this special veneration.

Piety and Instruction

Fortunately, there is more information available about an altarpiece in Florence, which contained several episodes from the lives of Cosmas and Damian, including the Miracle of the Black Leg (Ill. 11 page 60). A closer look may give some idea of the way in which works like these functioned and how, therefore, they should be seen.

In the course of 1442, brother Giovanni from Fiesole, now generally known as Fra Angelico, finished a large altarpiece for the church of the Dominican convent of S. Marco in Florence. The Dominicans had been mendicants since the foundation of the order in the twelfth century and did not have enough money to rebuild and restore the dilapidated complex of S. Marco, which their colleagues of the Sylvestrine order had abandoned in 1418. Most of the costs were therefore met by Cosimo de' Medici, a prominent Florentine banker as well as one the most influential political persons in the city. He also paid for Fra Angelico's large altarpiece, which was set up on the high altar of the church, opposite the entrance, and was dedicated on January 6th, 1443.

The main panel of this altarpiece (now in the San Marco Museum, Florence) shows the Holy Virgin Mary with the Christ child, sitting on a throne flanked by angels and saints (Ill. III page 24). On her left side stand Dominican and Franciscan saints, and on her right St. Mark, St. John the Evangelist and St. Lawrence. In front of them are two kneeling saints: Cosmas and Damian. These saints have not been included at random: the mendicant saints obviously refer to the Dominican monks, while St. Mark was the titular saint of the convent and its church. Sts John and Lawrence were the patron saints of respectively Cosimo de' Medici's father Giovanni and his brother Lorenzo. The two saints at the foreground refer to Cosimo himself. Both saints were doctors, *medici*, and therefore patron saints of the Medici-family. One of them, moreover, is called Cosmas or, in Italian, Cosimo. The inclusion of the Medici-related saints served as a demonstration of the piety of the Medici family members, in particular Cosimo who had sponsored the altarpiece, but also as an expression of their wealth and, by implication, power.

Under the main panel was originally a row of eight smaller panels – the so-called *predella*-paintings (*predella*, Italian, means step or dais). Unfortunately, they have been removed in later times and are now dispersed over several museums. They show various episodes from the life of Cosmas and Damian, according to the account in the *Golden Legend*. The last scene (now in the S. Marco Museum, together with the main panel), originally on the outer right corner, shows the Miracle of the Black Leg. Just like the saints in the main panel, the subjects of the *predella*-scenes had not been selected at random. On the most obvious level, they refer to the Medici family and to Cosimo in particular. On a different level, however, they serve as an example of Christian living for all observers, but especially for the Dominican monks. In the main panel, St. Mark is standing with an open bible, which he holds just above the head of St. Cosmas. The page on which it is opened contains the episode from the sixth chapter of his gospel, where – as related before – Christ sends forth his disciples two by two, charging them to take nothing for their journey, to cast out devils and to heal the sick. The *predella*-scenes illustrate how Sts Cosmas and Damian fulfill this charge. Thus they are seen healing Palladia and refusing to accept a reward;[2] preaching to the proconsul Lysias and freeing him from a devil; being tortured to death (cf. *Matthew* 10:18-22 and *Mark* 8:34-37); and finally carrying on their healing works after their death, through such miracles as the healing of the cancerous leg. All these acts correspond perfectly to the aims of the Dominican order: poverty, preaching, and an ardent faith.

One may wonder, of course, if the monks at S. Marco's were able to recognize that these scenes from the lives of Cosmas and Damian were meant to express the ideals of the Dominicans' mission. Most probably, they did indeed understand it, as seems to be borne out by the specific selection of *predella* scenes. The chosen episodes largely follow the account of the *Golden Legend*, but not totally. For instance, only one posthumous act is represented, while the other two have been skipped. This particular selection corresponds to the readings from the *Golden Legend* that were yearly recited to the monks during matins (pre-dawn office) on September 27, the (Roman Catholic) feast of Sts Cosmas and Damian.[3] The monks, in other words, were familiar with the choice of acts as presented in Fra Angelico's altarpiece, and over the years they had become trained to consider them as exemplary deeds that were particularly relevant for Dominicans.

Truth and Tradition

The San Marco-altarpiece may have been exceptional in its sophistication. Not all altarpieces and *predella*-scenes were so carefully thought over and the various parts were not always so well adjusted to each other. Around 1434, for example, Fra Angelico painted an earlier version of the Miracle of the Leg (Ill. 10 page 59), for the *predella* of an altarpiece of which the various scenes formed a less coherent whole. Yet the choice of Cosmas and Damian-scenes can still be explained in reference to Cosimo de' Medici and his family. The same is true for most of the other Cosmas and Damian-scenes that were made in Florence during the fifteenth century.

These Florentine pictures shed light on another point: the importance of artistic traditions. It is obvious that the painters and sculptors, rather than studying medical procedures in a hospital, looked at each others' works and took over such things as the scheme of the composition and the

---

2 Damian, however, was so weak as to accept a modest gift from Palladia, after she had urgently insisted that he take it. In Fra Angelico's painting, this 'reward' consists of a little dish with food.

3 In 1969, the feast of Cosmas and Damian was moved to September 26.

way the miraculous surgery is performed: without any loss of blood and with hardly any tools or assistance from others. Within these various artistic traditions, the paintings of Ambrosius Francken (Antwerp, 1593) (Ill. 40 page 103) and Gian Battista Tinti (Parma, 1594) (Ill. 42 page 105) stand out for their (relative) 'realism'. Varying traditions, however, do not explain everything. The function of a work of art is an important factor as well. Ambrosius Francken's painting (Ill. 40 page 103) looks more like an actual amputation because the patrons were members of the Barbers' and Surgeons' Guild in Antwerp. They not only wanted to dedicate an altarpiece to their patron saints in the local cathedral, but at the same time wanted to give a demonstration of their surgical skills. Gian Battista Tinti had to make a painting for the local brotherhood of Sts Cosmas and Damian. He showed the saintly brothers as professional doctors who are in close contact with the heavenly hosts.

Yet not even such paintings as those by Francken and Tinti should be seen as 'truthful' documents of contemporary surgical practice. Three woodcut illustrations from sixteenth century handbooks for surgeons may illustrate this further: one from Hans von Gersdorff's *Feldtbuch der Wundartzney* (Strasbourg, 1517), the other from Walther Hermann Ryff's *Die grosse Chirurgei* (Frankfurt a. M., 1545) and the third from Theophrastus Paracelsus's *Opus Chyrurgicum.... Wund und Artzneybuch* (Frankfurt a.M., 1566) (Ill. VI-VIII pages 27-29). All three show a patient who is more than conscious of what is happening to him. A surgeon with a saw is cutting the leg and many other tools are close at hand. Profusely streaming blood is caught in a barrel, even though a bandage has been tied tightly around the leg, so as to cut off the bloodstream. In the woodcut from Ryff, moreover, someone is covering the patient's eyes, so that at least he will not have to see what is happening to him. The actual sawing and cutting is done by men in short tunics. This indicates that they are practicing surgeons, to be distinguished from university-trained physicians, who would wear long, academic gowns. In the print from Ryff, the man covering the eyes of the patient and holding a book may be an academic doctor, while the two other men are practicing surgeons.

Although all three prints may also fail in accuracy, they undoubtedly give a more 'realistic' idea of the way legs were amputated, than illustrations of the Miracle of the Black Leg do. However, it was never the artists' aim to show explicitly the upsetting details involved in this kind of surgery. Moreover, the story in the *Golden Legend* relates that the saints performed their miracle while the man was asleep. This means that there was no need to show a patient writhing with pain and, more importantly, that some of the mystery of the event had to be expressed. The Florentine painters of the fifteenth century did this by showing how the sick man calmly sleeps on, while Cosmas and Damian do not perform any fearsome surgery, but simply take off the affected leg and replace it by the healthy one. In this way, the dream-like aspect and the mystery of the miracle have been preserved. Most Spanish painters put more emphasis on the supernatural aspect of the incident. They added angels who serve as a sort of operating room assistants, while Cosmas and Damian perform their miraculous healing just as smoothly and cleanly as in Italian paintings. In the pictures by Fernando del Rincón de Figueroa (Ill. 21 page 70) and Andrés Sánchez de Oña (the so-called Master of the Balbases, Ill 22 page 71), the surgical skills of the saints consist of making a blessing gesture; the latter even made the incident seem more the celebration of mass than the healing of a sick person.

Yet the artists often added 'medical instruments', so as to create the impression that even in the case of the miraculous surgery there were true (former) doctors at work. This was, of course, in close correspondence with the account of the *Golden Legend*, where the brother saints appeared to the sick man 'bringing salves and surgical instruments'. It was even more in accordance with pictorial traditions and 'trends'. Especially in the case of Spanish and North Italian representations of the miracle (as, for instance, the beautiful fresco in Ferrara, Ill. 18 page 67) the artists betrayed the influence of Northern European paintings, where depictions of interiors often contained all kinds of domestic details, rendered with much attention and precision. There is abundant evidence that Northern European paintings were much admired and avidly collected in Italy and Spain. Native painters from these countries tried to meet this admiration by adopting Northern European elements in their works. Thus, the rooms where Cosmas and Damian are performing their miracle often look like fifteenth century Flemish interiors, with all their paraphernalia: copper bowls, pewter pitchers and glass vessels. None of these actually resemble real medical instruments like those on the foreground of the three woodcuts showing the actual amputation of a leg. This again demonstrates how exceptional Ambrosius Francken's painting from ca. 1590 is. (Ill. 40 page 103) The Northern artist must have included actual surgical tools to satisfy explicit demands of his professional patrons, the members of the Antwerp Guild of Barbers and Surgeons.

Details and Particulars

It may be revealing, after these general observations, to highlight a few aspects in detail and focus on some individual illustrations.[4]

The painting in Vienna (Ill. 44 page 107) is the most accurate illustration of the account in the *Golden Legend*. Just as in the text, there is actually no leg replaced. Cosmas and Damian carved out the rotten flesh (*caro putrida*) of the affected leg, so as to replace it with the healthy flesh of a recently died man from Ethiopia. The continuation of the legend's text is a little confusing, as it relates that Cosmas and Damian subsequently took the Moor's hip (*cox*) and placed in the white man's body. The Vienna painting shows in the background that Cosmas and Damian did indeed not amputate the leg of the Ethiopian man. Instead, they carved a part out of it and implanted this piece into the white man's leg. Consequently, the white man has kept his own, white lower leg, and only his upper leg (including the hip) has become black.

At variance with the legend's text, all the other illustrations show that the white man's leg is actually supplanted. Already the earliest examples, from the fourteenth century, contain this

---

4 Illustrations made in Spain are discussed in the contribution by Carmen Fracchia.

anomaly. They were at the start of a visual tradition that apparently had a stronger impact on the artists of the following generations than the letter of the legend's text. There is, however, no consistency as to which leg was affected or how it was replaced. Some artists made it the right leg, others the left. Jaume Huguet, in a *predella* painting from 1460 for the church of Santa María de Terrasa, near Barcelona, confused left and right (Ill. 15 page 64). In the background, Cosmas and Damian are amputating the dead Ethiopian's right leg. On the foreground, however, they are substituting a left leg! In some pictures, it is only the part under the knee that is restored, in others the complete leg, up to the hip. In Pesellino's *predella* picture from c. 1440-45, it seems to be the leg including the hip that is replaced (Ill. 12 page 61). Very difficult to illustrate was the fact that the miracle took place while the affected man was asleep – which means, supposedly, during the hours of darkness. In most pictures, however, it is daytime. Mariotto di Nardo, in the early fifteenth century, seems to have been the first to introduce a sleeping person, as an indication that the event occurred during the night (Ill. 5 page 54). The presence of a sleeping person turned out to be a successful motif, which would be repeated by many other artists. Bicci di Lorenzo found a clever solution in his *predella* picture from 1429 (Ill. 09 page 58). He showed that Cosmas and Damian perform their miracle in a room where it is light, even though outside it is clearly night.

Usually, the man whose leg is restored is not aware of what is going on. In accordance with the text of the legend, he is asleep. Even in the pictures where he is awake – or seems to be so – he quietly submits to the knife. A number of artists have put the dead man from Ethiopia next to the bed where the sick man is lying, even though the corpse was (and remained) in the cemetery of the church of St Peter-in-Chains. By including him in the bedroom, however, they tried to make the story extra clear and express the miraculous nature of the event. The white man has now been happily equipped with a healthy black leg, while the Moor's dead body is foisted off with a putrid white limb.

In general, the pictures show a tendency to suppress the upsetting aspects involved in the amputation and replacement of a limb. Blood is conspicuously absent in all of them. Some pictures do hint at loss of blood and, by implication, some experience of pain, but none of it is actually shown. The early sixteenth century painting in Stuttgart, for instance (Ill. 28 page 77), shows how both the white and the black leg have been amputated with a straight, clear cut. Consequently, the black leg seamlessly attaches to the white man's stump. Only a thin red edge where the leg has been cut off and a bowl under the bed give an inkling of the (possible) flow of blood. The amputated white leg in the foreground does not show any of the 'rotten flesh' (*caro putrida*) that the text of the legend mentions, and seems in still good condition. Three angels serve as operating room assistants, holding aspersoriums (holy water sprinklers) instead of medical instruments. Apart from the angels, all these aspects are also true for the fresco in Ferrara, from 1476 (Ill. 18 page 67). The absence of blood, pain and suffering adds to the sense that what is being performed is not an ordinary surgical treatment, but a miracle.

Only a few paintings show that the amputated leg was (in the words of the legend) 'totally consumed by a cancer'. In a late painting from 1691, (Ill. 54 page 117) in the church of Sts Cosmas and

Damian in Uboldo, Stefano Maria Legnani (usually called il Legnanino) makes an angel specifically point out how badly affected the leg is. The much earlier painting by Paolo Bontulli in Tazza, from 1516, (Ill. 32 page 95) shows the amputated limb prominently on the foreground, looking seriously corroded by black wounds. Cosmas and Damian, accompanied by three other men, are on the point of attaching the fresh leg, simply – it seems – through the act of prayer. Their medical instruments are lying in front of the patient's bed, like a sort of still life. The miniature painted around 1465, by Girolamo da Cremona, also shows a seriously putrified leg, on a plinth on the foreground (Ill. 17 page 66). Cosmas and Damian stand near it, their medical instruments in their hands. Behind them, the aftermath of the miracle is illustrated. Witnesses stare in amazement at the white man's healthy black leg, while in the right background bystanders seem just as surprised ogling the Moor's grave. On the left, surrounded by clouds and angels, God the Father blesses the scene.

Two paintings deserve special attention for the remarkable way in which they depict the miraculous healing. The first one is the painting by the Master of the Legend Scenes in Vienna (Ill. 44 page 107). Several of its unusual features have already been mentioned, and one of the most special is that Cosmas and Damian are not in it! On the left side, the sick man is lying in bed, having just woken up and inspecting his healthy but black upper leg with a candle. In the middle of the picture, he is out of bed and lifts up his clothes to show his friends what has happened. In the background, people gather around the grave of the dead Moor, who is indeed missing a part of his upper leg. Some of them have wrapped their clothes around their nose, as a sign that the corpse is not as fresh as the *Golden Legend* tells. Cosmas and Damian are nowhere to be seen. The same is true of the two accompanying scenes, which illustrate the legend of the wife saved from the devil. There, Cosmas and Damian are not visible either, even though their presence is certainly implied (Ill. IX page 30). This absence indicates that the original ensemble, to which these pictures belonged, must have contained a separate panel, or perhaps statuettes, that prominently displayed the saints. At the same time, the painter may have considered it an artistic challenge to depict a miraculous healing without showing anything supernatural.

The second painting that deserves special attention is the left wing of an altarpiece from 1593, by Ambrosius Francken (Ill. 40 page 103). It is the most 'realistic' of all representations. One of the reasons why it shows the amputation of a limb in a quite explicit way has already been mentioned. Its patrons of the Barbers' and Surgeons' Guild not only wanted to dedicate a painting to their patron saints, but also desired a picture that would demonstrate their surgical skills. Francken seems to have served them well. He shows both saints dressed as practicing surgeons in short tunics, and not as academic doctors in long gowns. In the foreground, he added real surgeons' tools. The operation is not taking place in a private bedroom, but in a hospital room where other patients are also undergoing surgery and examination. Any sense of something supernatural is absent. Cosmas and Damian are not even recognizable by a halo around their head, and contrary to all the other representations, the patient is painfully aware of what is being done to him. Obviously, Francken's sources of inspiration were not earlier representations of the Miracle of the Leg. To satisfy his patrons' request for a 'realistic' depiction, he must have turned to treatises on surgery. Apparently he found a very useful example in Paracelsus's *Opus Chyrurgicum .... Wund und Artzneybuch* from 1566 (Ill. VIII page 29).

Changing Beliefs and Traditions

Most of the representations of the Miracle of the Black Leg were made in the fifteenth and sixteenth century. After ca. 1580, their number decreased considerably. That was largely the result of growing skepticism towards exceedingly wondrous miracles like the replacement of the affected leg. Spurred on by criticism from the Protestants and the decrees of the Council of Trent (1545-1564), the Catholic Church took a more discriminating look at the credibility of the saints and their many legends. Although the veneration of time-honored saints did not totally disappear, saints like the giant Christopher or the dragon killer George were steadily pushed to the background. Around 1580, such prominent cardinals as Caesar Baronius and Joannes Molanus considered their legends superstitious. From then on, these saints appear less often in works of art. The same fate hit spectacular miracles such as those performed by St. Nicholas. In the light of these developments, it is understandable that the Miracle of the Black Leg was less frequently represented. It did not totally disappear, but in those few cases when it was depicted, it followed new standards. The paintings by Gian Battista Tinti from 1594, (Ill. 42 page 105) by Stefano Maria Legnani (il Legnanino) (Ill. 54 page 117) and by an anonymous artist in Grazzano Visconti (Ill. 57 page 120) stress other aspects than the pictures from before ca. 1580. They show the sky opening up above the two saints, exposing St Mary and the heavenly host. The clouds revealing this celestial glory give the paintings a visionary quality, in which Cosmas and Damian no longer seem to be the ones who perform the miracle, but just medical agents who act through divine assistance. This novel way of considering saints and presenting them in art is sometimes foreshadowed in the sixteenth century, as for instance in the painting in Pegola di Malalbergo (Emilia-Romagna, Italy), by Bartolomeo Ramenghi (better known as 'il Bagnacavallo', 1484-1542) (Ill. 47 page 110). In general, however, it conforms to a trend in the seventeenth and eighteenth century, when saints were no longer perceived as miracle workers, but as visionaries who communicate with the divine.

The number of pictures of the Miracle of the Black Leg after the eighteenth century is small. With increasing skepticism towards faith in general and miracles in particular, this is understandable. Consequently, 'modern' representations no longer serve the function of inspiring the viewers to reverence and devotion. They are now created to indicate, for instance, that a certain building or institution is named after (or was originally dedicated to) Sts Cosmas and Damian, or that it has a medical function. Examples are the glass stained window by Christoph Stooss for the Medical Society in the canton of Zurich (1992), (Ill. 68 page 143), the medallion by Evariste Jonchère at the Nouvelle Faculté de Médicine in Paris (1953), (Ill. 70 page 145) the woodcut by Yves Alix (1890 – 1969) (Ill. 62 page 137) and the sculpture in wood by Tomasita J. Rodriguez in

Santa Fe (Ill. 76 page 151). Since the 1990's, there seems to have been a sudden increase of icon-like representations of the Miracle of the Black Leg in a (neo) Byzantine style. This 'revival' has exclusively happened in Greece and its adjacent regions (Ill. 72, 78-81 pages 147, 153-156). What makes this phenomenon so special and un-historical, is that pictures of the black leg never occured in this part of Europe. As we have seen, the specific detail of a black replacement leg was unknown to the Orthodox Church.

Interesting as modern representations of the miraculous healing may be, they spring forth from an entirely different background than the earlier pictures. They should be seen as individual works of art, and no longer as illustrations of the power of faith in accordance with the teachings of the Church. The legend of the Black Leg originated as the tale of a miracle performed by two of God's faithful devotees. Illustrations had to express this supernatural dimension visually. Since the miraculous aspect of the story is no longer believed, however, illustrations of it have necessarily acquired a different character. Instead of an expression of God's wondrous working through his saintly agents, they have become testimonies of the fascination with an extraordinary story from a credulous past.

Literature

Useful books and articles with general information on Sts Cosmas and Damian, their veneration and their iconography, are:

David-Danel, M.-L. 1958. *Iconographie des saints médecins Côme et Damien*, Lille.
David-Danel, M.-L. 1970. *Répertoire pour la France des lieux de culte dédiés aux saints Côme et Damien*. (from: *Mélanges de science religieuse* 23 (1966)-26 (1969), Lille).
Wittmann, A. 1967. *Kosmas und Damian. Kultausbreitung und Volksdevotion*, Berlin.

The veneration and iconography of Cosmas and Damian in Eastern Europe is the subject of:

Skrobucha, H. 1965. *Kosmas und Damian*, Recklinghausen (*Iconographia Ecclesiae Orientalis*).

A Greek version of the legend of Cosmas and Damian, older than the one in the Golden Legend, has been edited by:

Deubner, L. 1907. *Kosmas und Damian. Texte und Einleitung*, Leipzig. (reprint: 1980, Aalen).

The history and the meaning of the Miracle of the Leg are discussed by:

Fichter, G. 1968 . 'Das verpflanzte Mohrenbein - Zur interpretation der Kosmas-und-Damian-Legende', *Medizinhistorisches Journal* 3/2, 87-100.

The interpretation of Fra Angelico's S. Marco-altarpiece is fully discussed by:

Hood, W. 1993. *Fra Angelico at S. Marco,* New Haven/London, 97-121.

The quote from the Zardino de oration is after:

Baxandall, M. 1988. *Painting and Experience in Fifteenth Century Italy. A Primer in the Social History of Pictorial Style*, Oxford/New York, 2nd ed., 46.

An excellent study of the transformation of the iconography of Christian art after the Council of Trent is:

Mâle, E. 1932. *L'art religieux après le concile de Trente. Étude sur l'iconographie de la fin du XVIe siècle, du XVIIe, du XVIIIe siècle*, Paris.

Useful information on the history (not, unfortunately, on the iconography) of the altarpiece by Ambrosius Francken is presented by:

de Poorter, N. 1970. 'De kunstwerken van het Antwerpse barbiers- en chirurgijnsambacht', in: *Liber memorialis: 350 jaar Collegium medicum Antverpiense*, Antwerp, 123-36.

Information on the individual paintings can usually be found in the relevant museum catalogues and on several places on the internet.

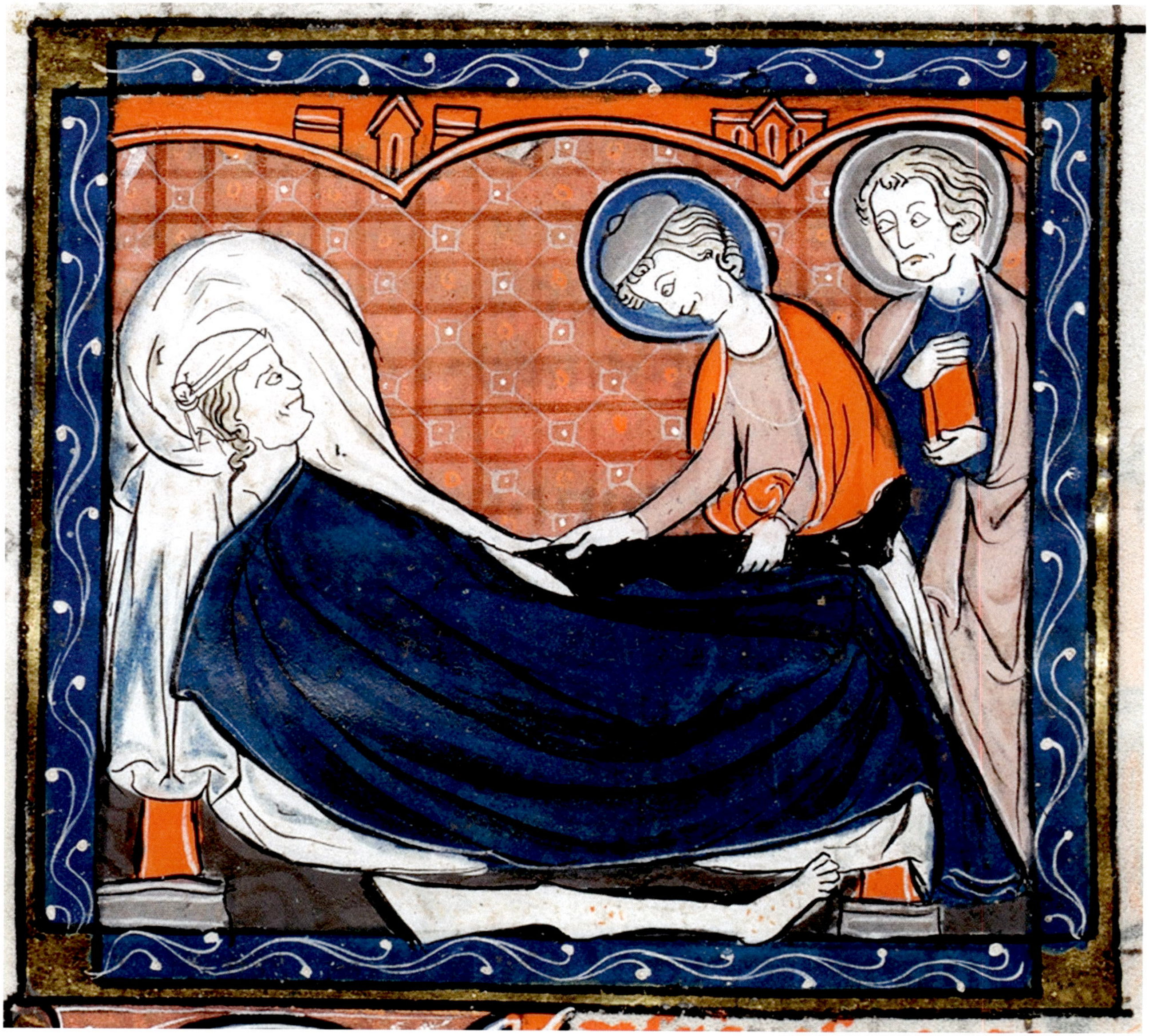

01. **Anonymous,** *illustration in manuscript, Legenda Aurea,* end 13th century. Henry E. Huntington Library, San Marino (U.S.A.).

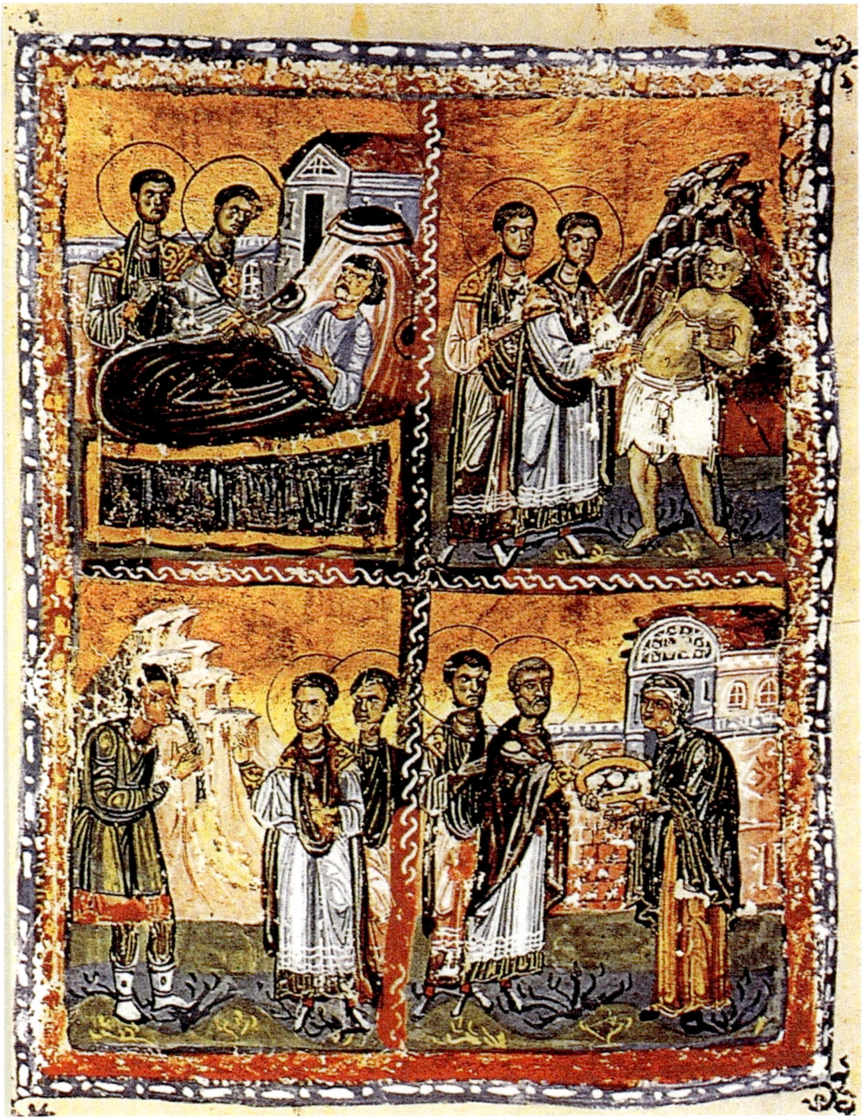

02. **Anonymous,** *illustration in manuscript,* 11th-12th century(?). Άγιος Παντελεήμων (Monastery of Saint Panteleimon), Athos (Greece).

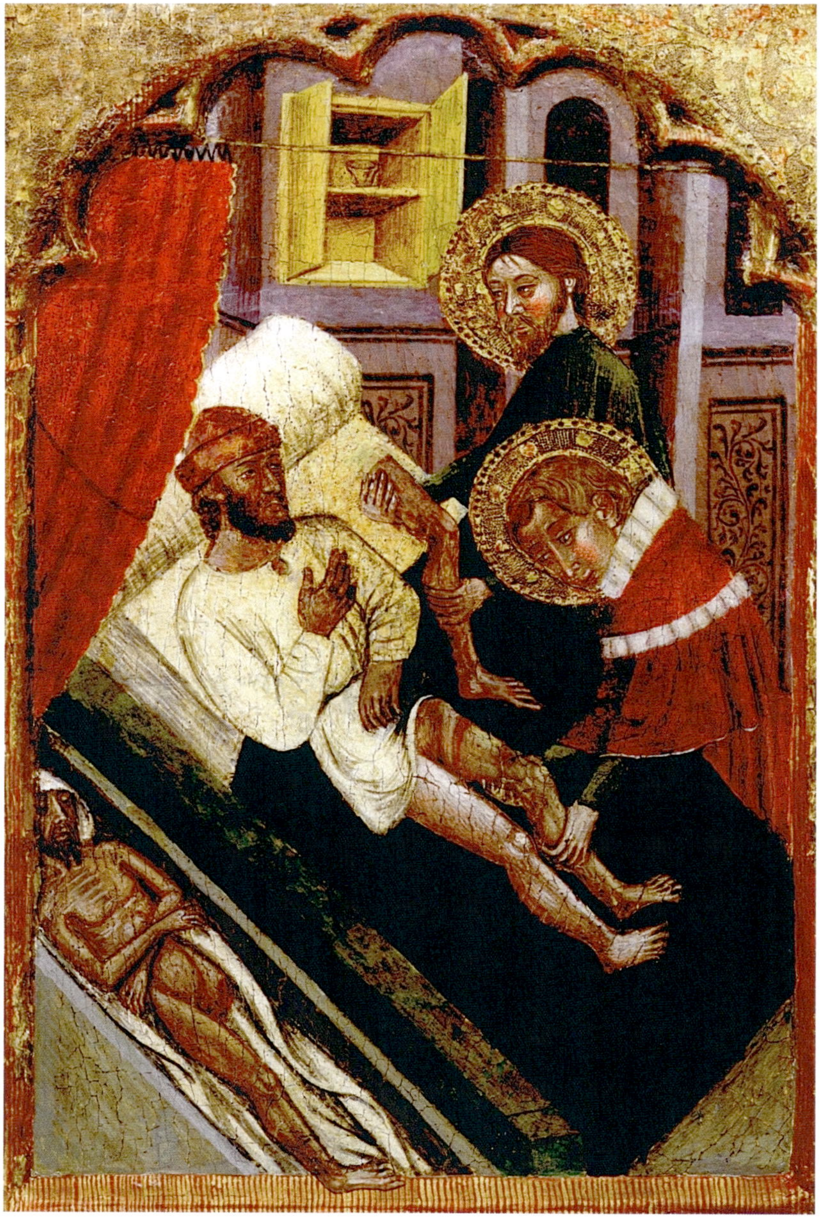

03. **“Master of Rubió”** active ca. 1351/52–1370/80, *panel*. Museo Arqueologico Episcopal, Vich (Spain).

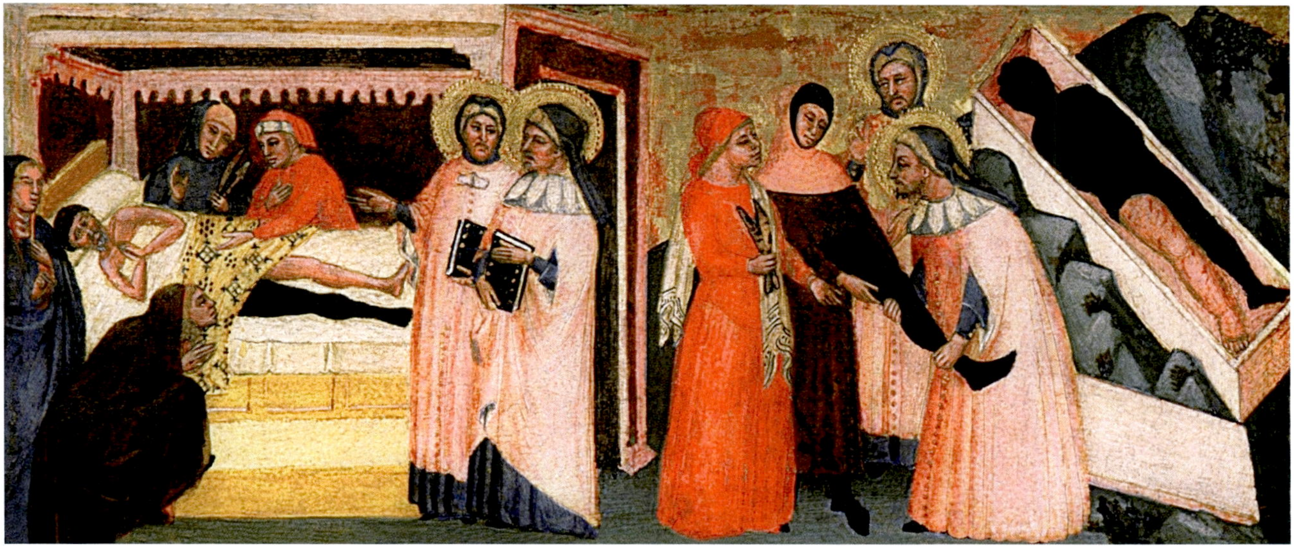

04. **"Master of the Rinuccini Chapel" (Matteo di Pacino?)** active 1350-1374 (1359-1375), *panel (predella scene).* 1370-1375 North Carolina Museum of Art, 'Gift of the Samuel H. Kress Foundation', Raleigh N.C. (U.S.A.).

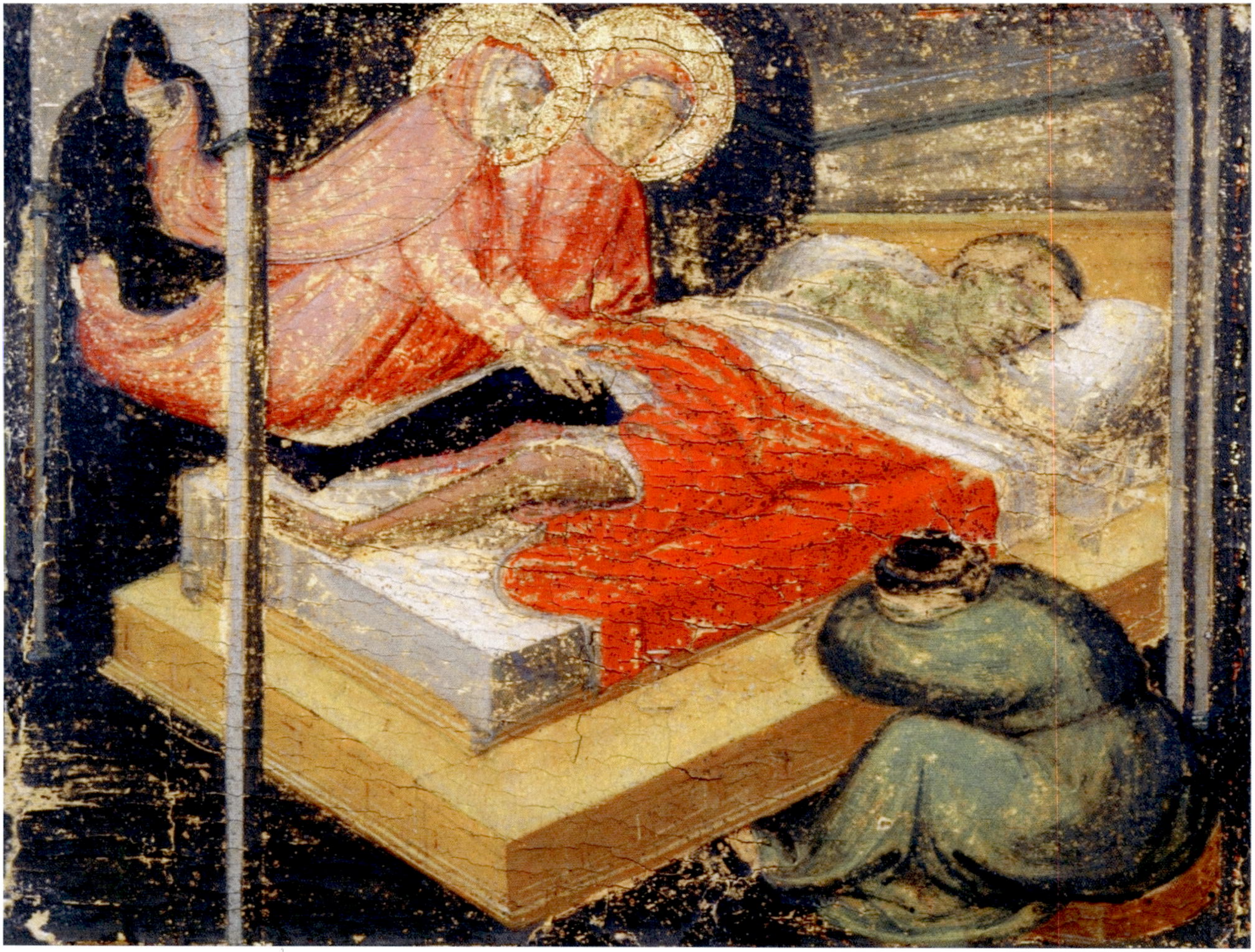

05. **Mariotto di Nardo,** (active 1394-1424), *panel (predella scene),* altarpiece for S.Croce, Florence.
Yale University Art Gallery, New Haven C.T. (U.S.A.).

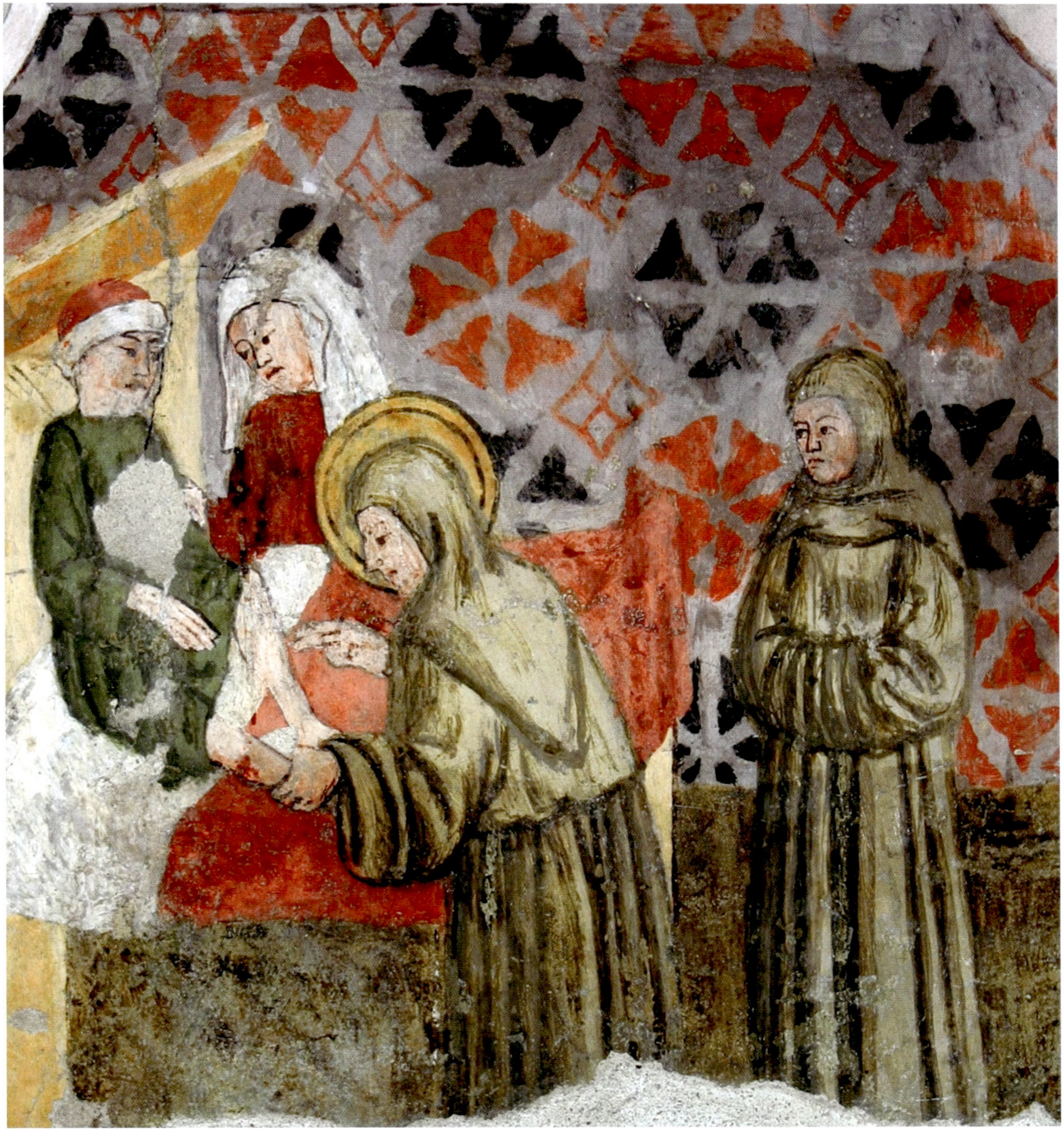

06. Anonymous, *fresco*, 14th century. S. Francesco, Deruta (Italy).

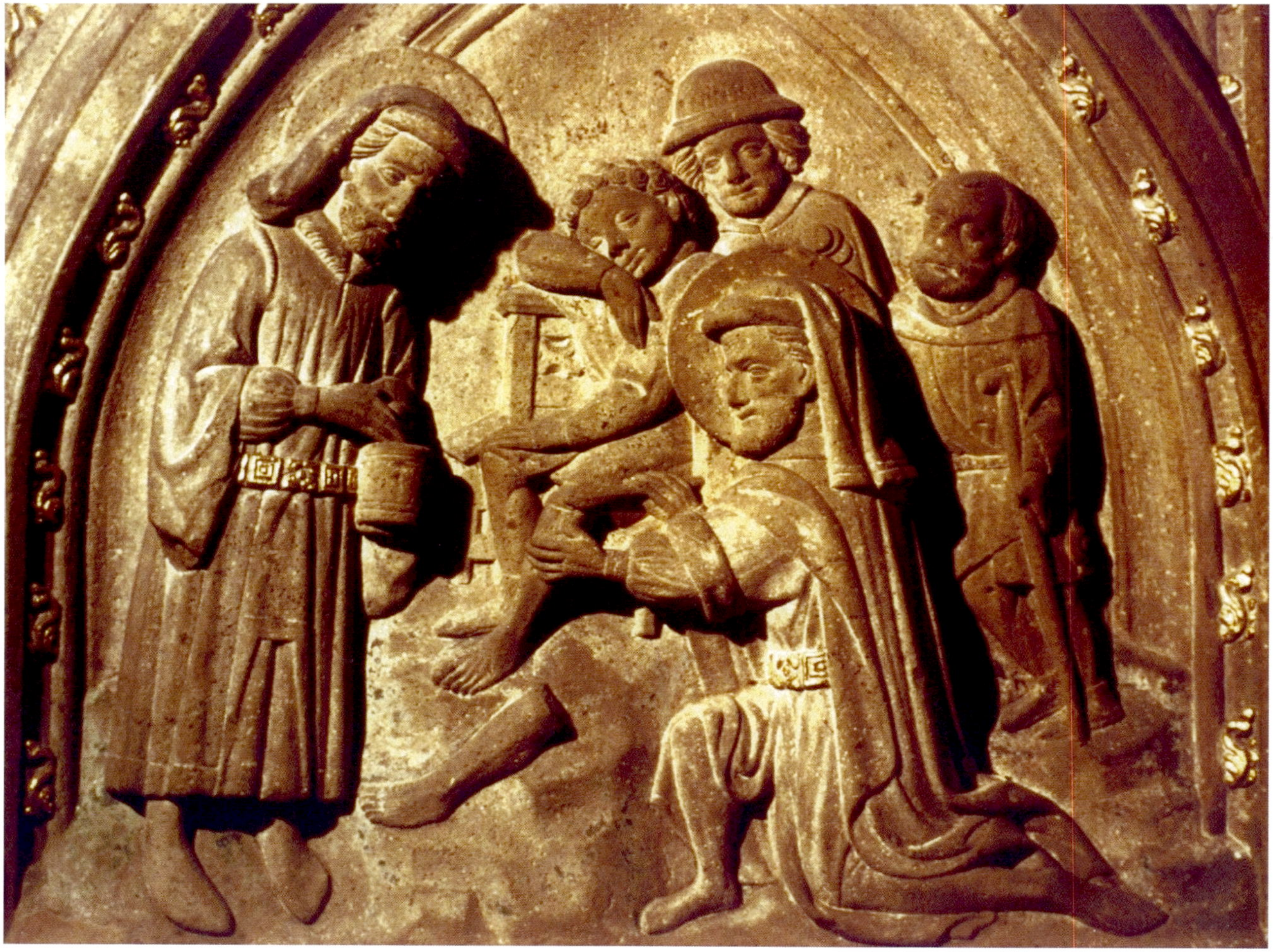

07. **Anonymous,** *sculpture in sandstone,* ca.1400. Dommuseum, Bremen (Germany).

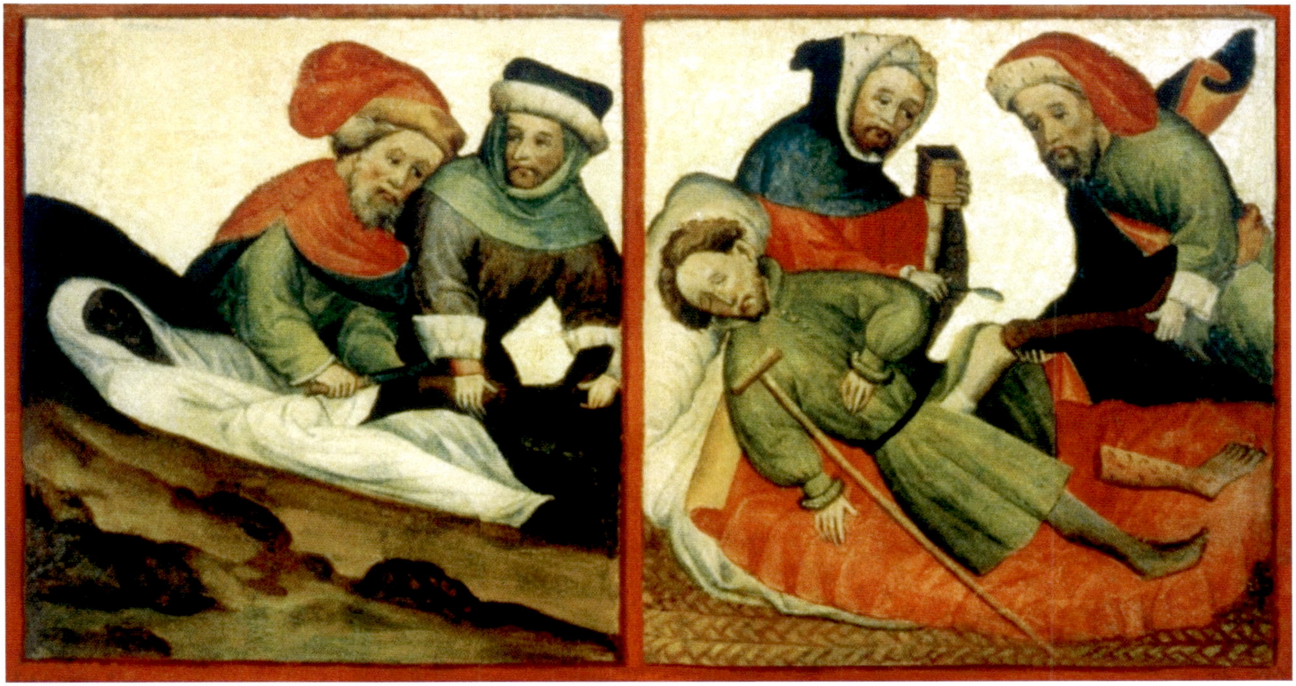

08. **Anonymous,** *painting inside reliquary,* 1402. St. Michaelkirche, München (Germany).

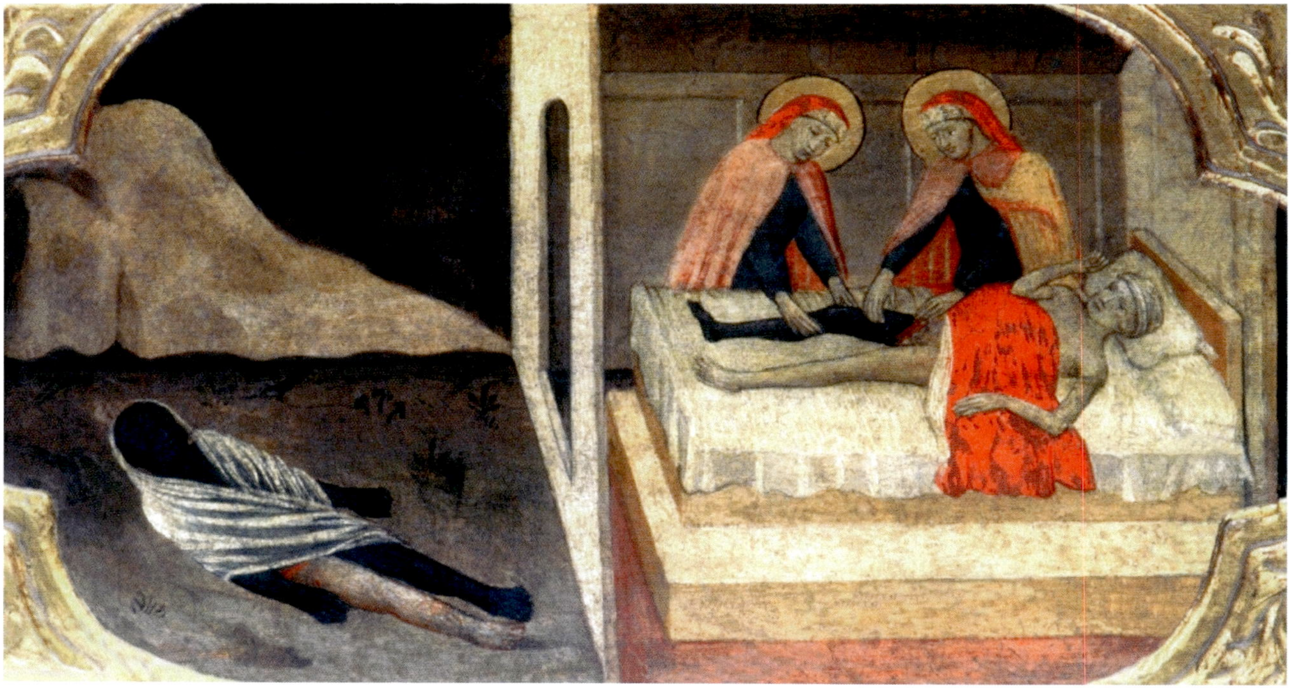

09. **Bicci di Lorenzo** (Florence, 1373-1452, Florence), *panel (predella scene)*, 1429. Basilica di Santa Maria del Fiore (Duomo), Florence (Italy).

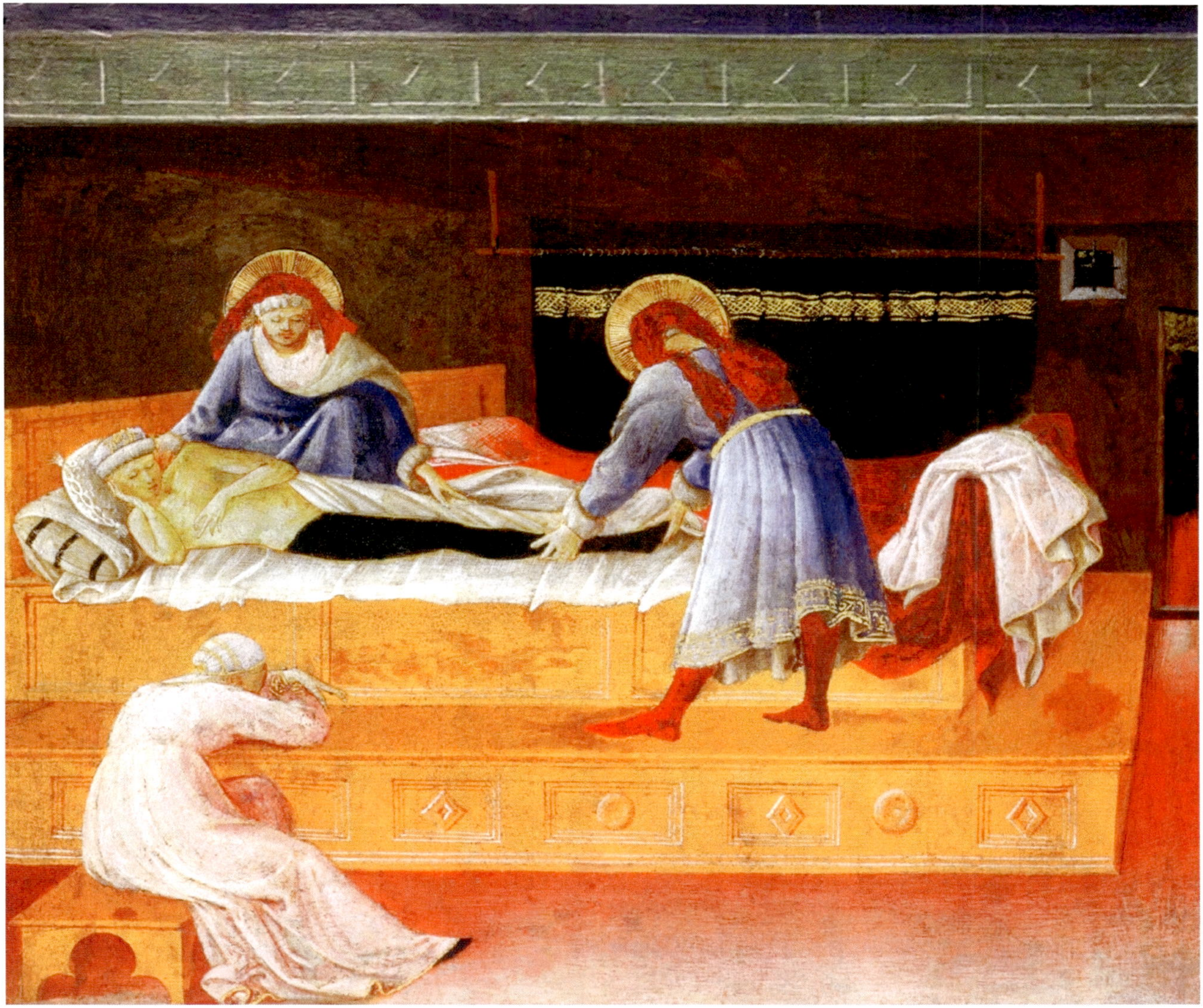

10. **Fra Angelico** (Rupecanina, ca. 1387-1455, Rome), *panel (predella scene)*, 1434. Kunsthaus Zürich, Zürich (Switzerland).

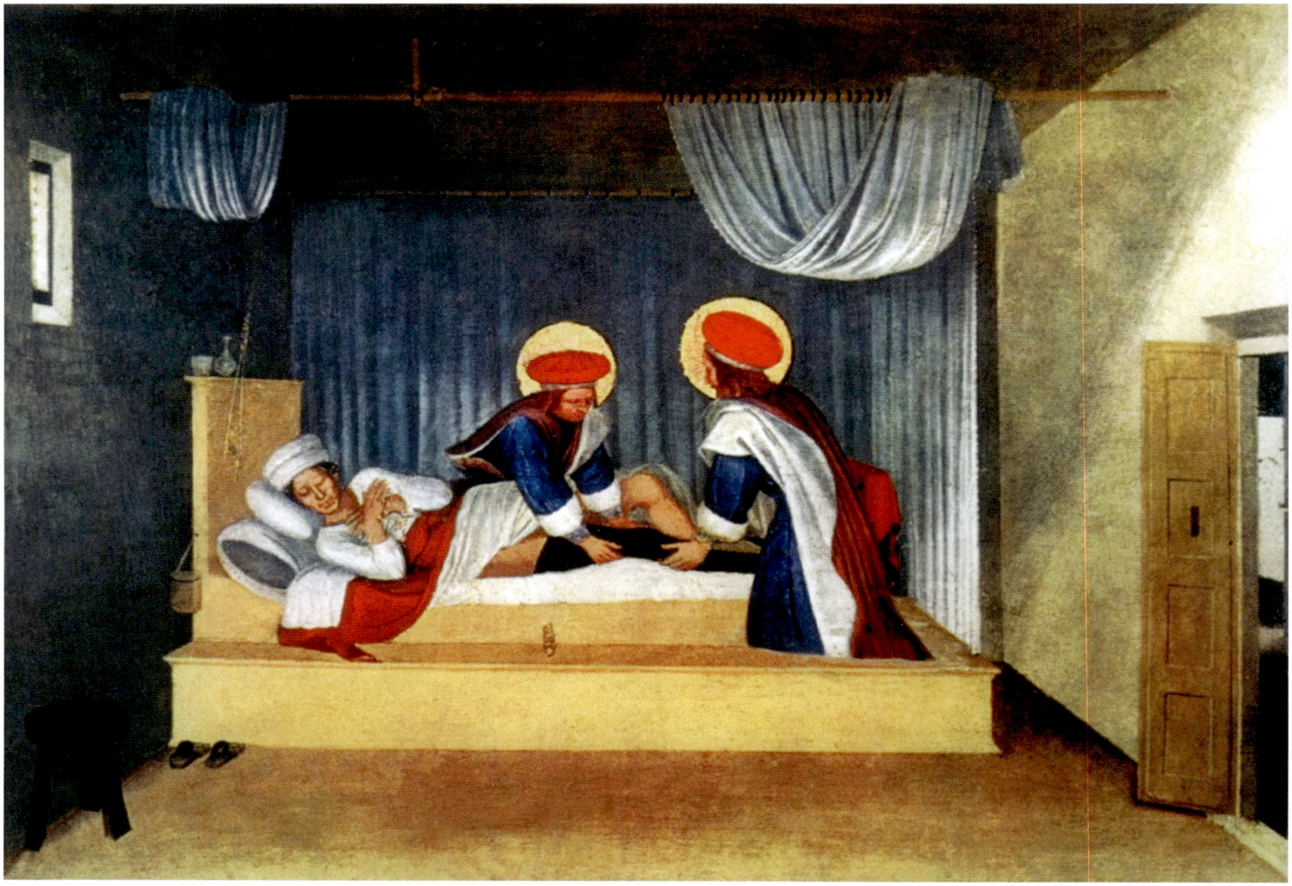

11. **Fra Angelico** (Rupecanina, ca. 1387-1455, Rome), *panel (predella scene),* 1442. Museo di S. Marco, Florence (Italy).

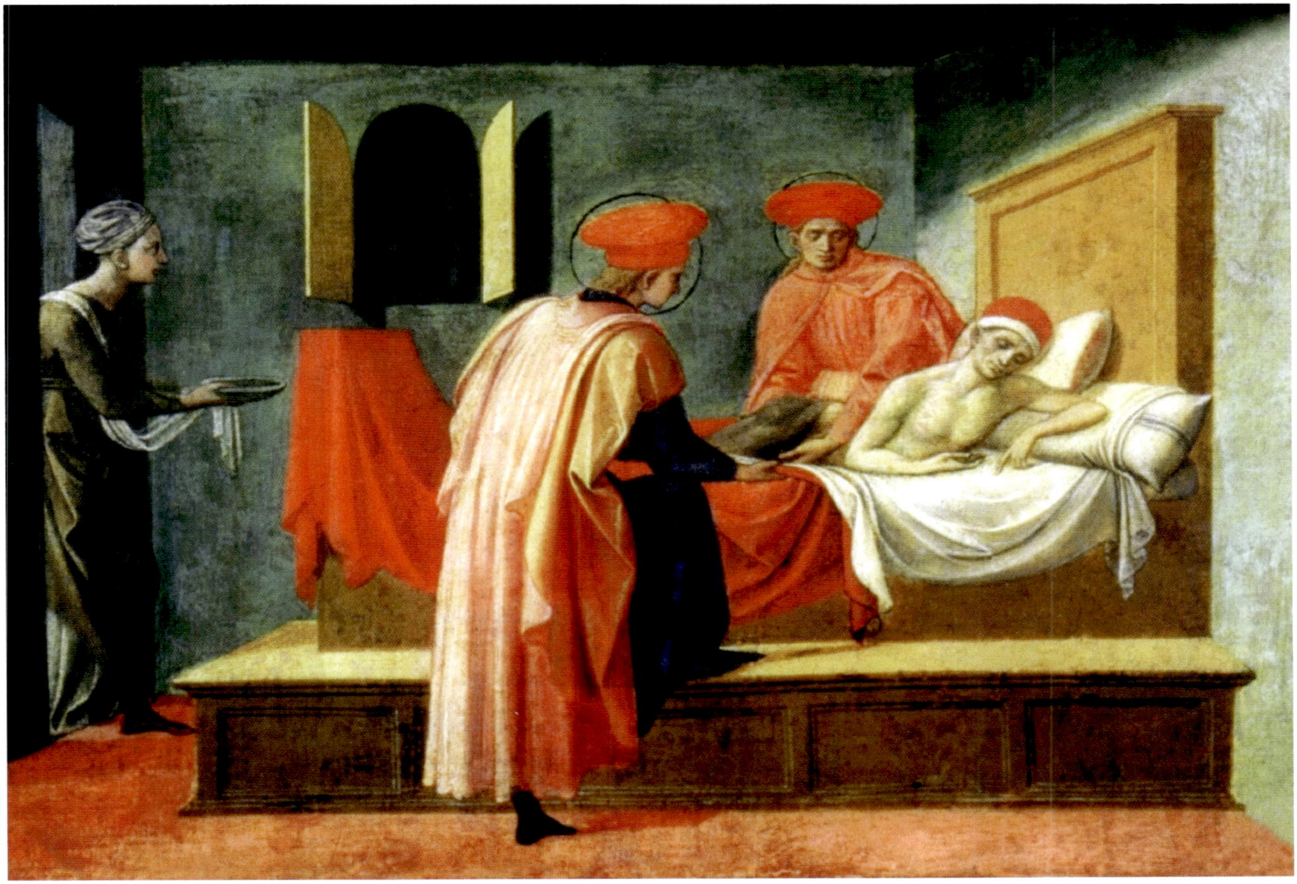

12. **Francesco Pesellino** (Florence, ca.1422-1457, Florence), *panel (predella scene)*, 1440/45. Musée du Louvre, Paris (France).

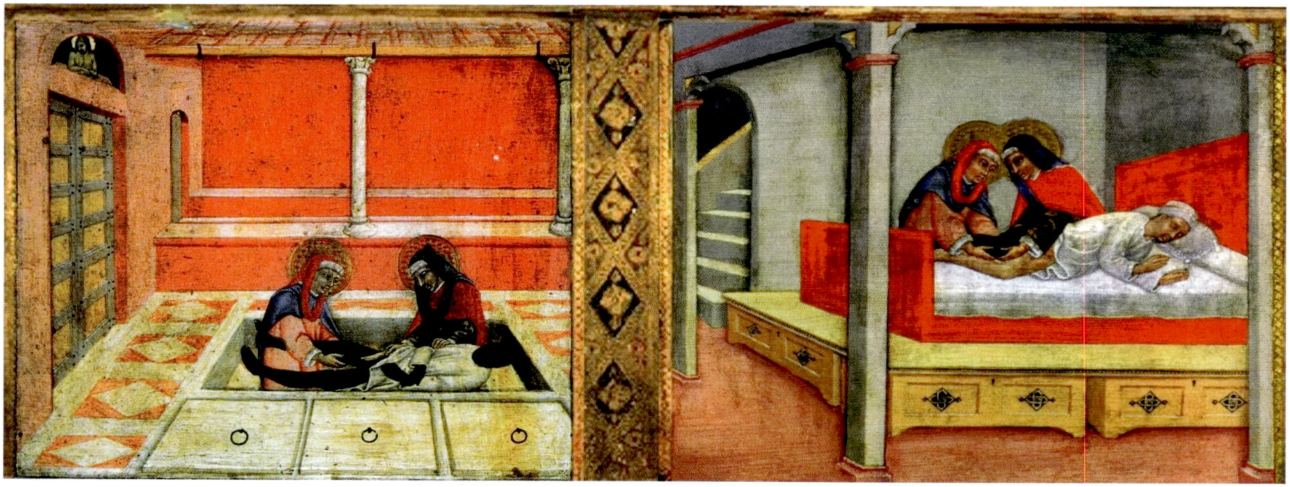

13. **Sano di Pietro** (Siena, 1406-1481), *panel (predella scene)*, 1447. Pinacoteca Nazionale di Siena, Siena (Italy).

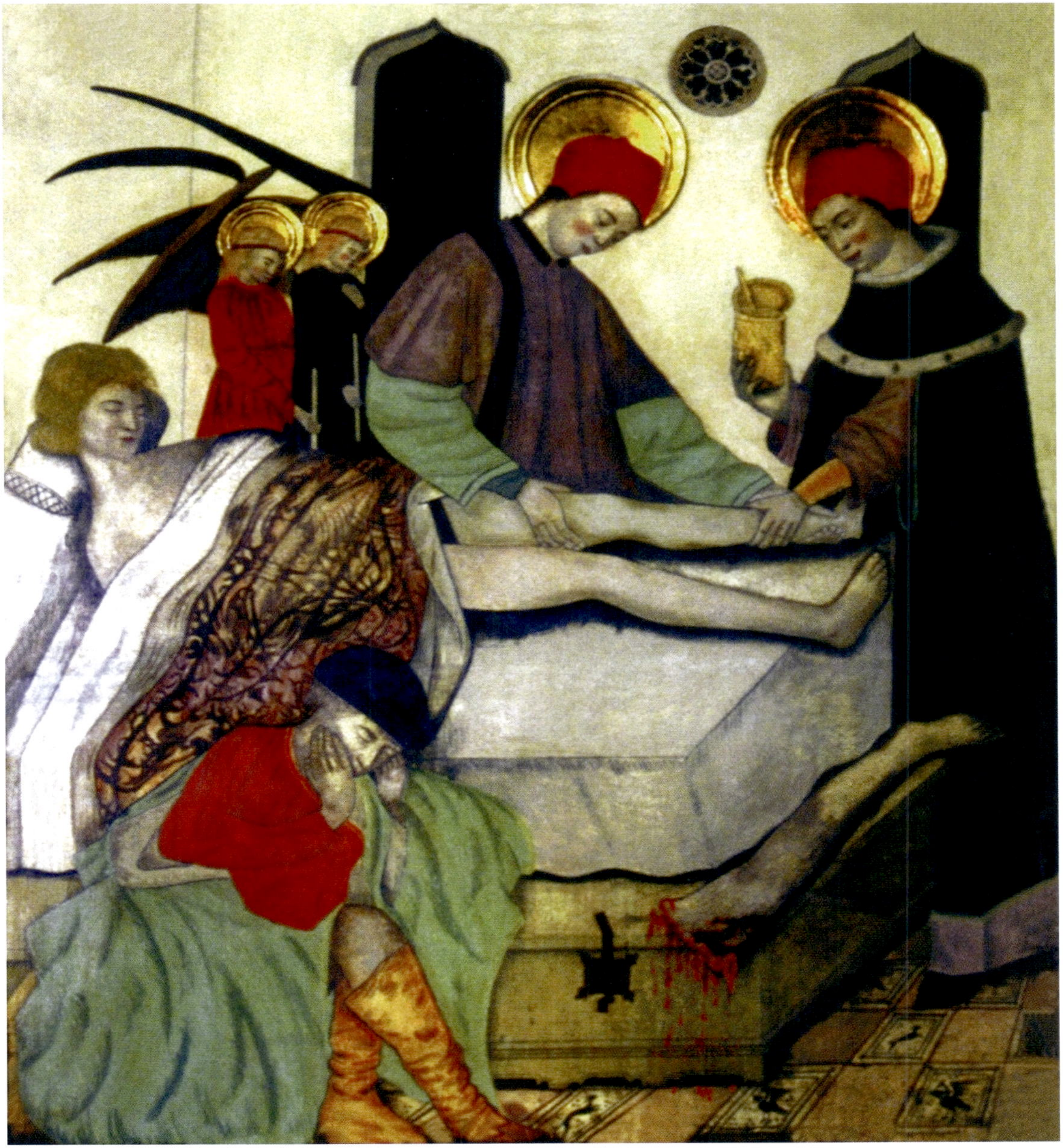

14. **Miguel Nadal** (ca. 1419-1492), *panel of altarpiece,* ca. 1454. Catedral de la Santa Cruz y Santa Eulalia, Barcelona (Spain).

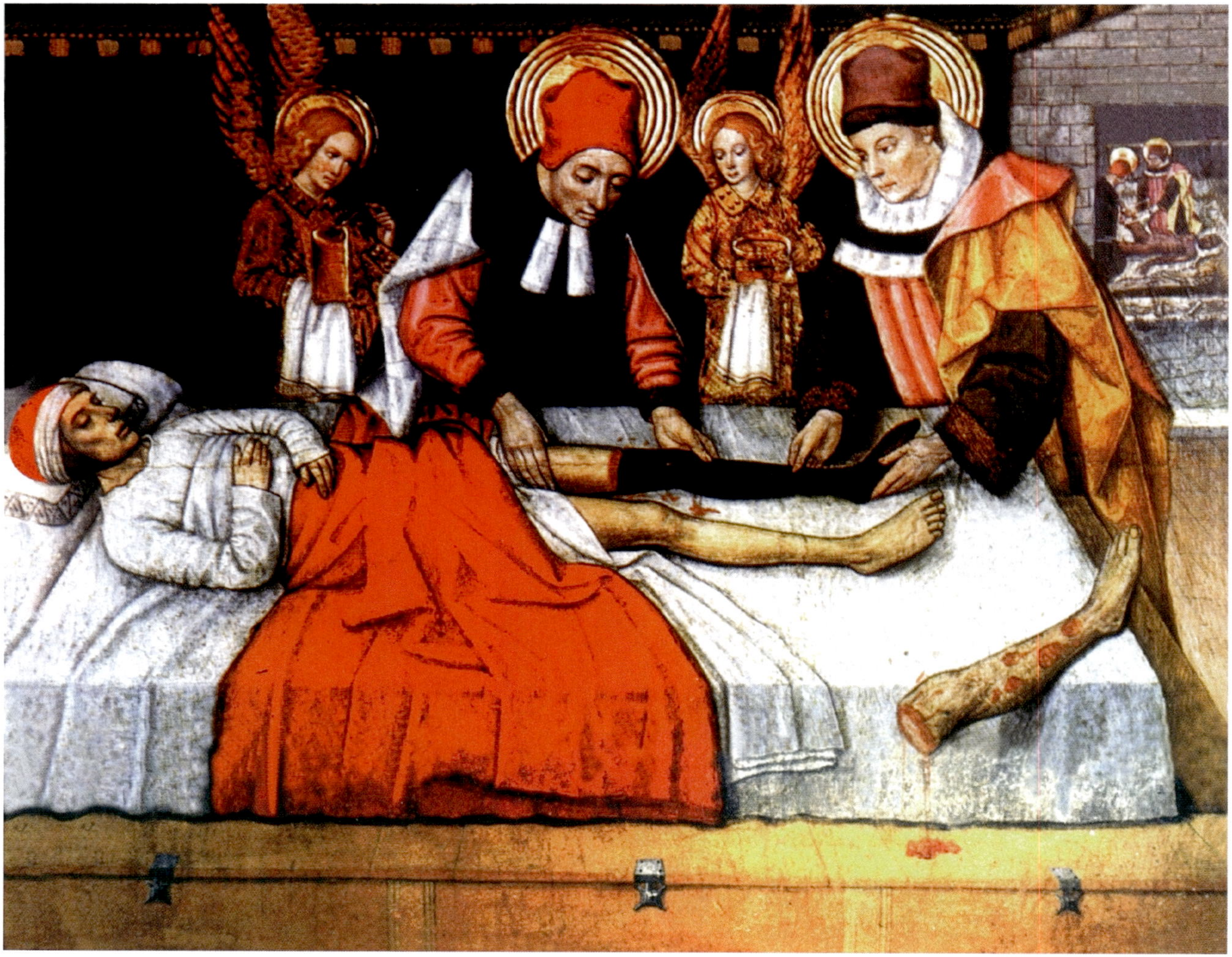

15. Jaume Huguet (Valls, ca. 1412-1492, Barcelona), *panel (predella scene)*, 1460. S.Maria (originally for S.Miguel),Terrassa (Spain).

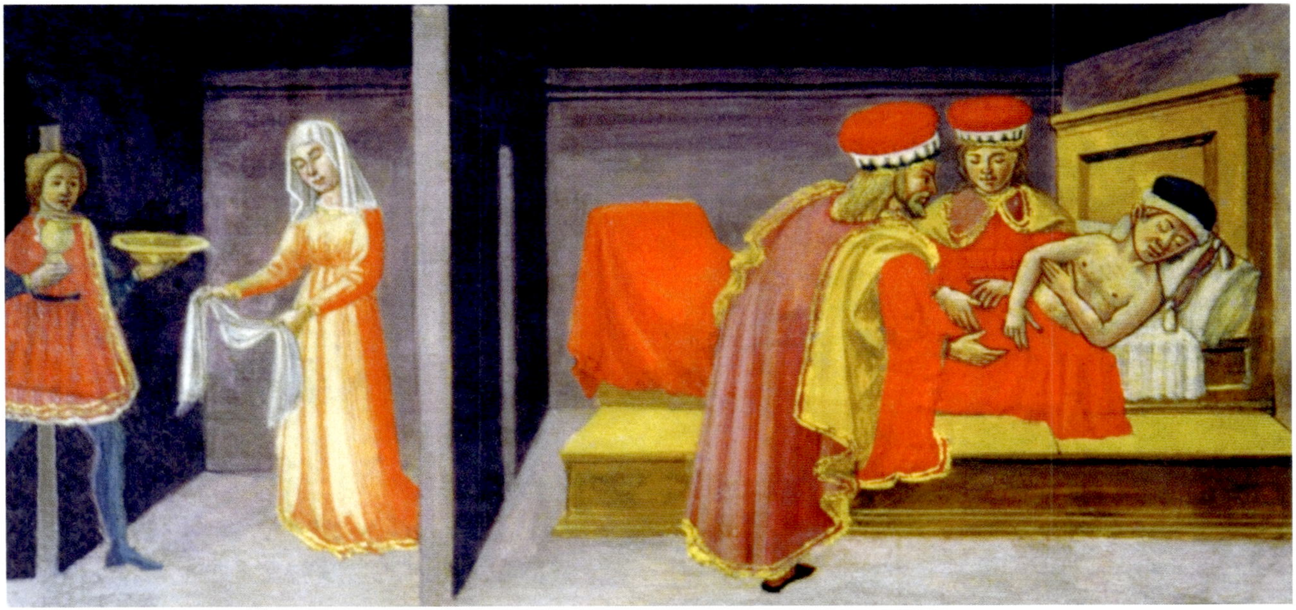

16. **Giusta d'Andrea** (1440-1496), *panel (predella scene).* S.Domenica (SS. Jacopo e Lucia de Foris portam), San Miniato, (Italy).

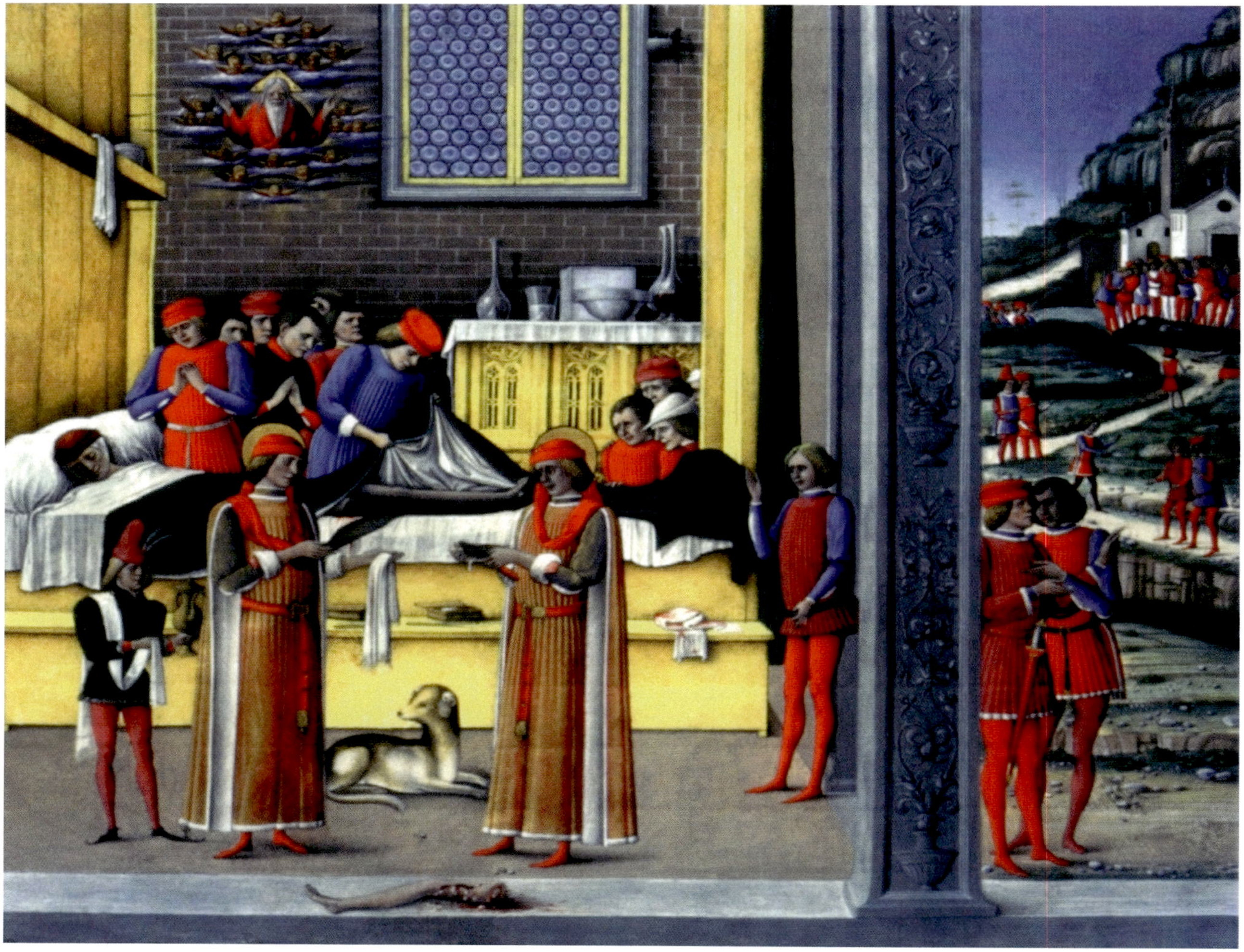

17. **Girolamo da Cremona,** active 1451-1483, *illustration in antiphonarium of Sts. Cosmas and Damian,* 1465.
Burlington House ms.450, fol. Ir, London (UK).

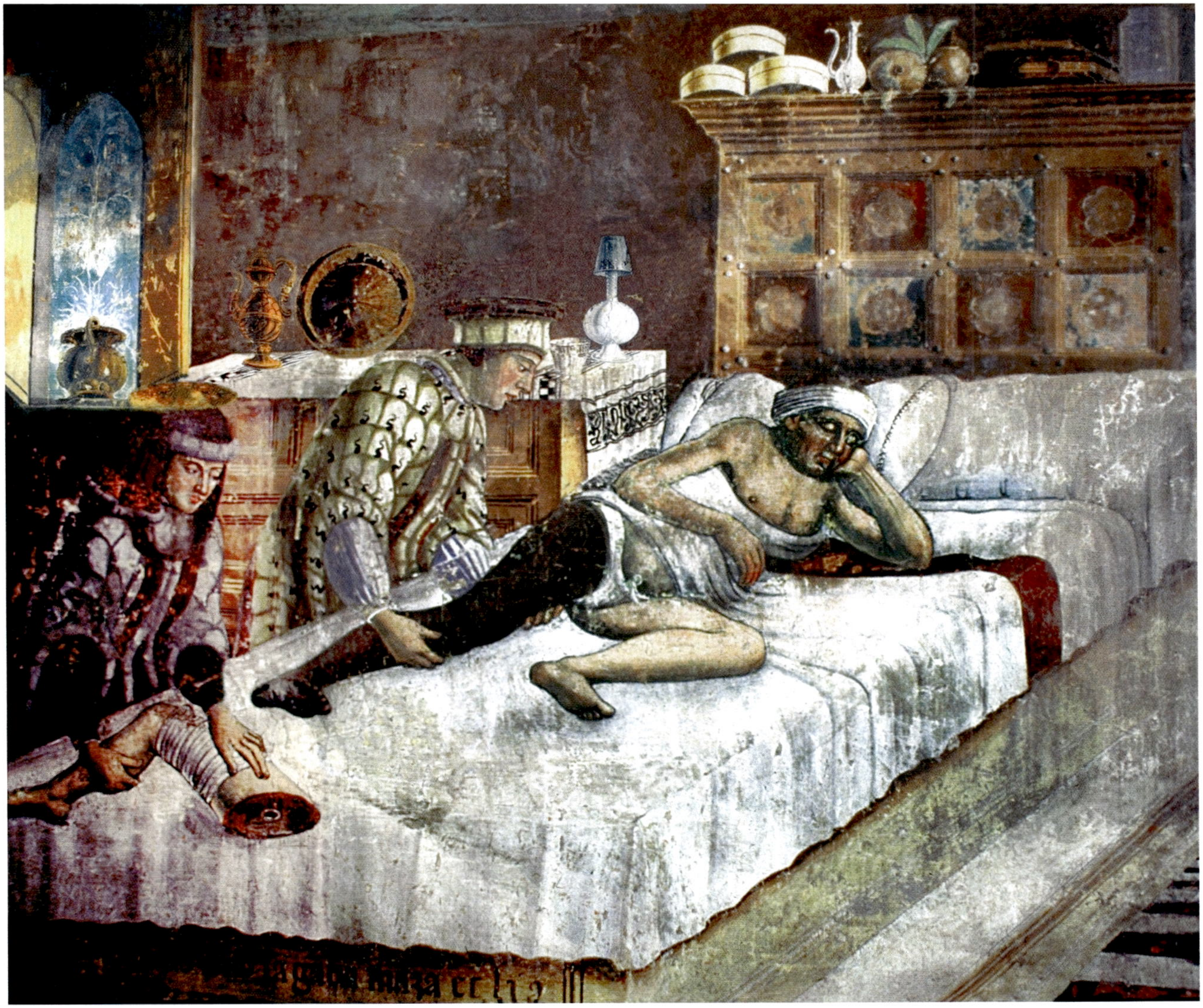

18. **Anonymous,** *fresco*, 1476. S.Paolo, Ferrara (Italy).

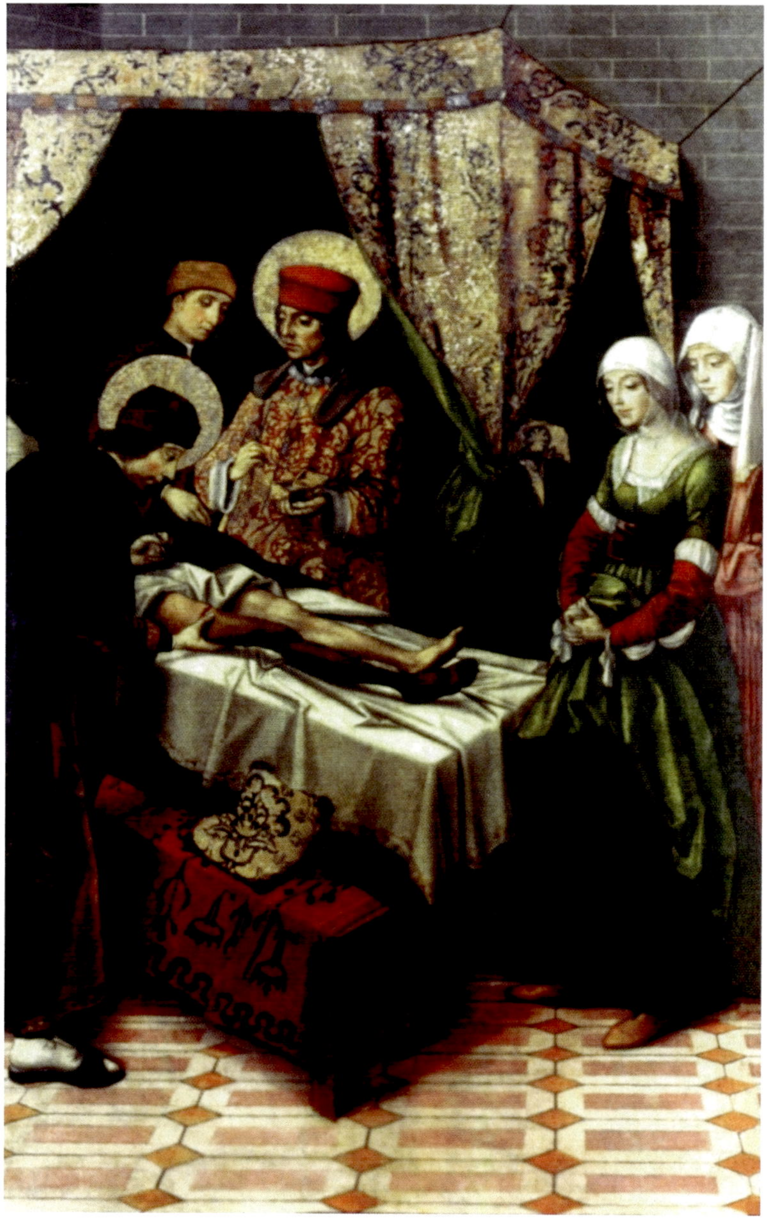

19. **Pedro Berruguete** (Paredes de Nava, ca. 1445-1504, Palencia), *painting on wood,* 1496. Colegiata, Covarrubias (Spain).

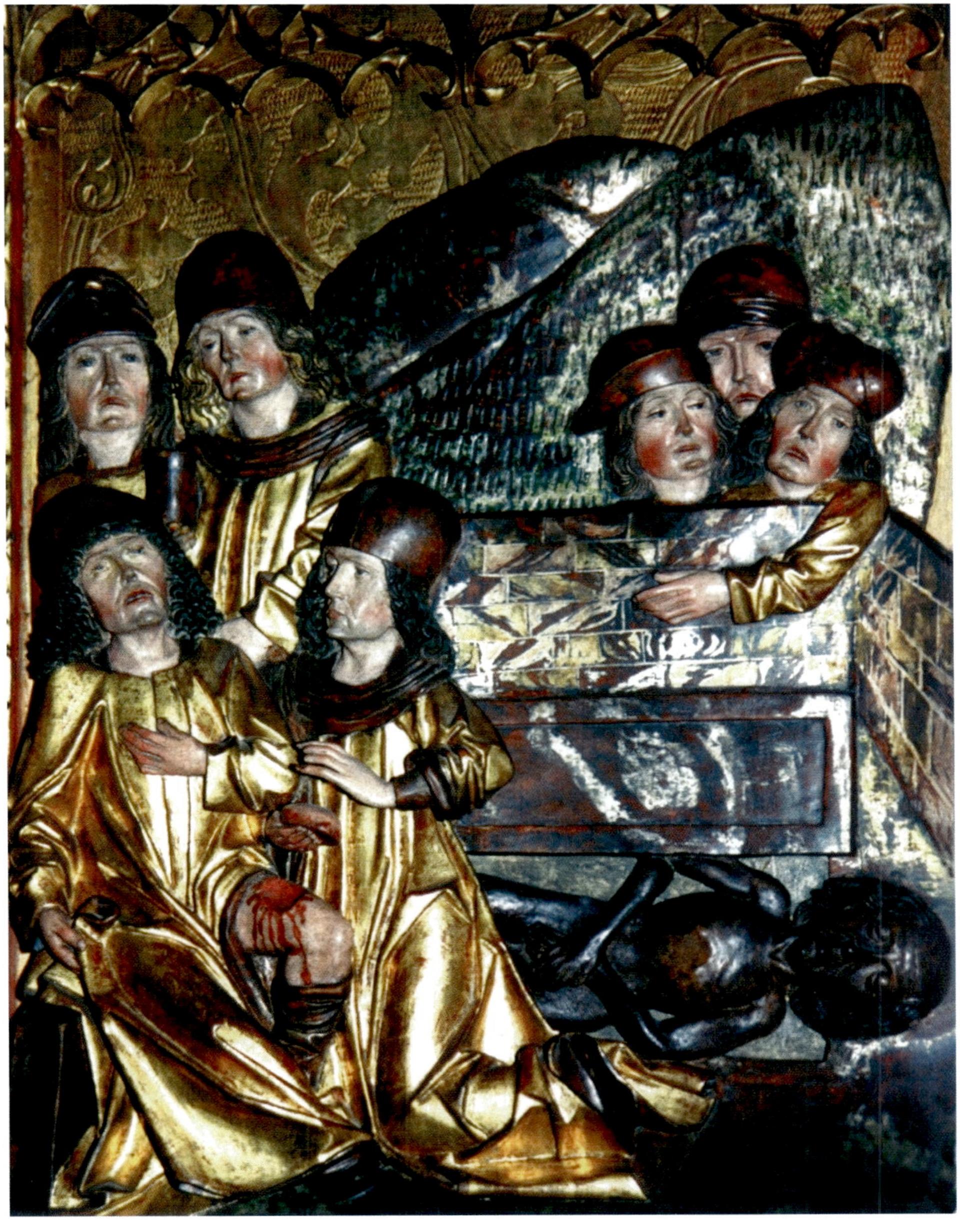

20. **Simone da Tesido (Simon von Taisten)** (1450(?)-1515(?)), *panel of altarpiece, polychrome woodcarving (from Sonnenburg).* Stadt Museo für Grafik, Brüneck (Italy).

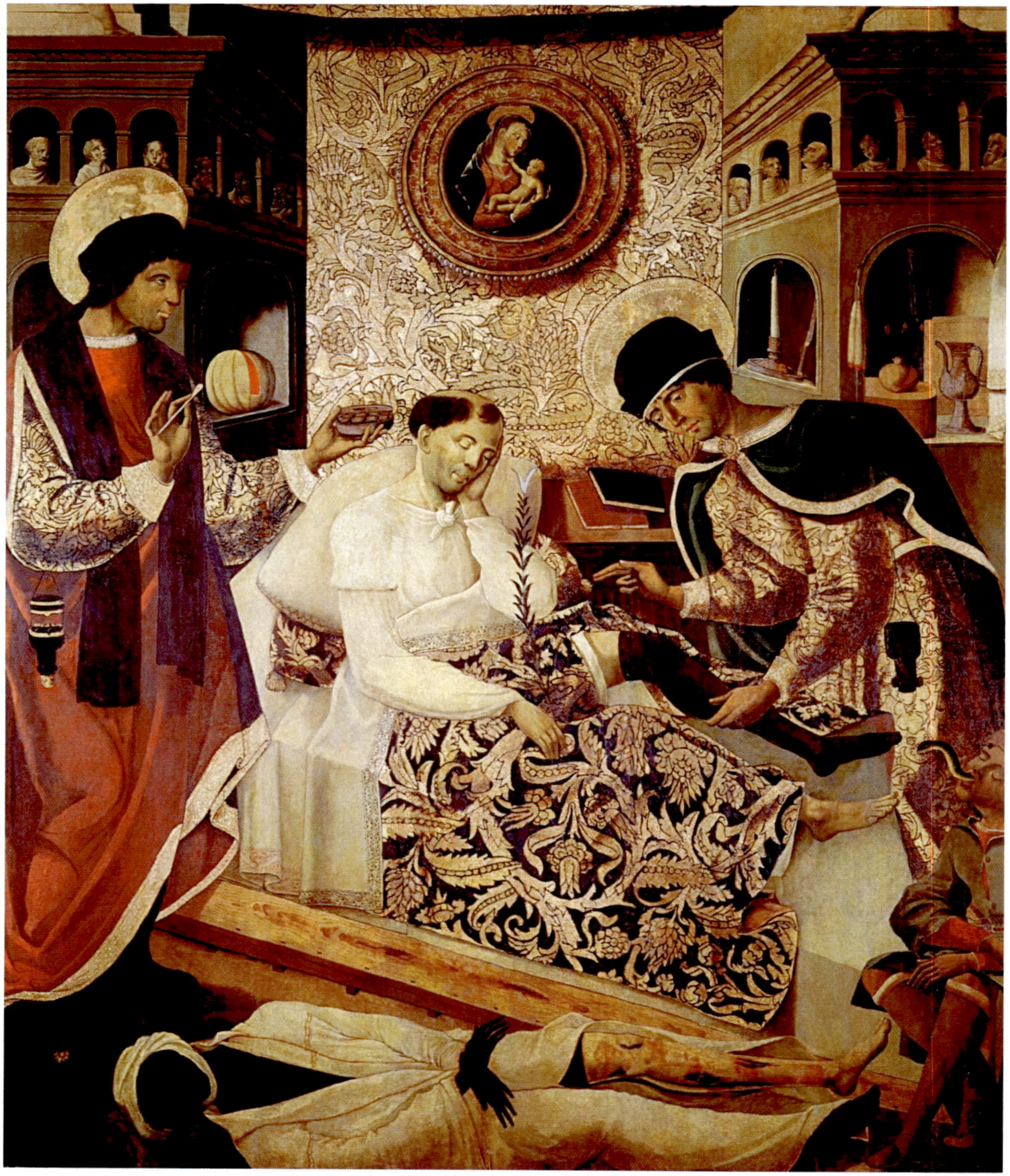

21. **Fernando del Rincòn de Figueroa** (Guadalajara, 1460-1529, Guadalajara), active 1491-1518, *painting.*
Museo Nacional del Prado, 'Derechos reservados © Museo del Prado – Madrid', Madrid (Spain).

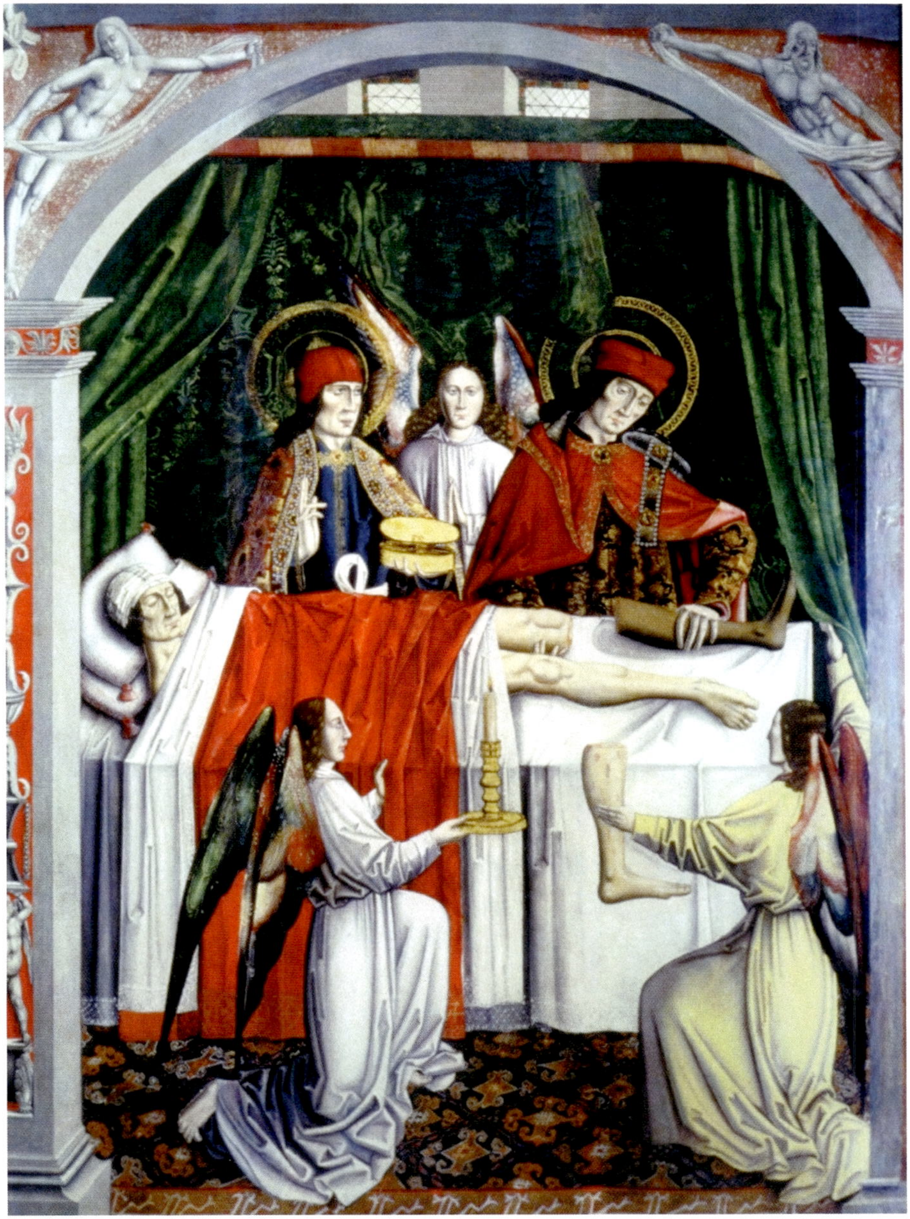

22. **Andrés Sánches de Oña (Master of Los Balbases)**, active in Burgos 1484-1510, *painting*, 1495. Originally in the royal church of Cosmas and Damian in Burgos, now in Wellcome Museum of Medical Science, London (UK).

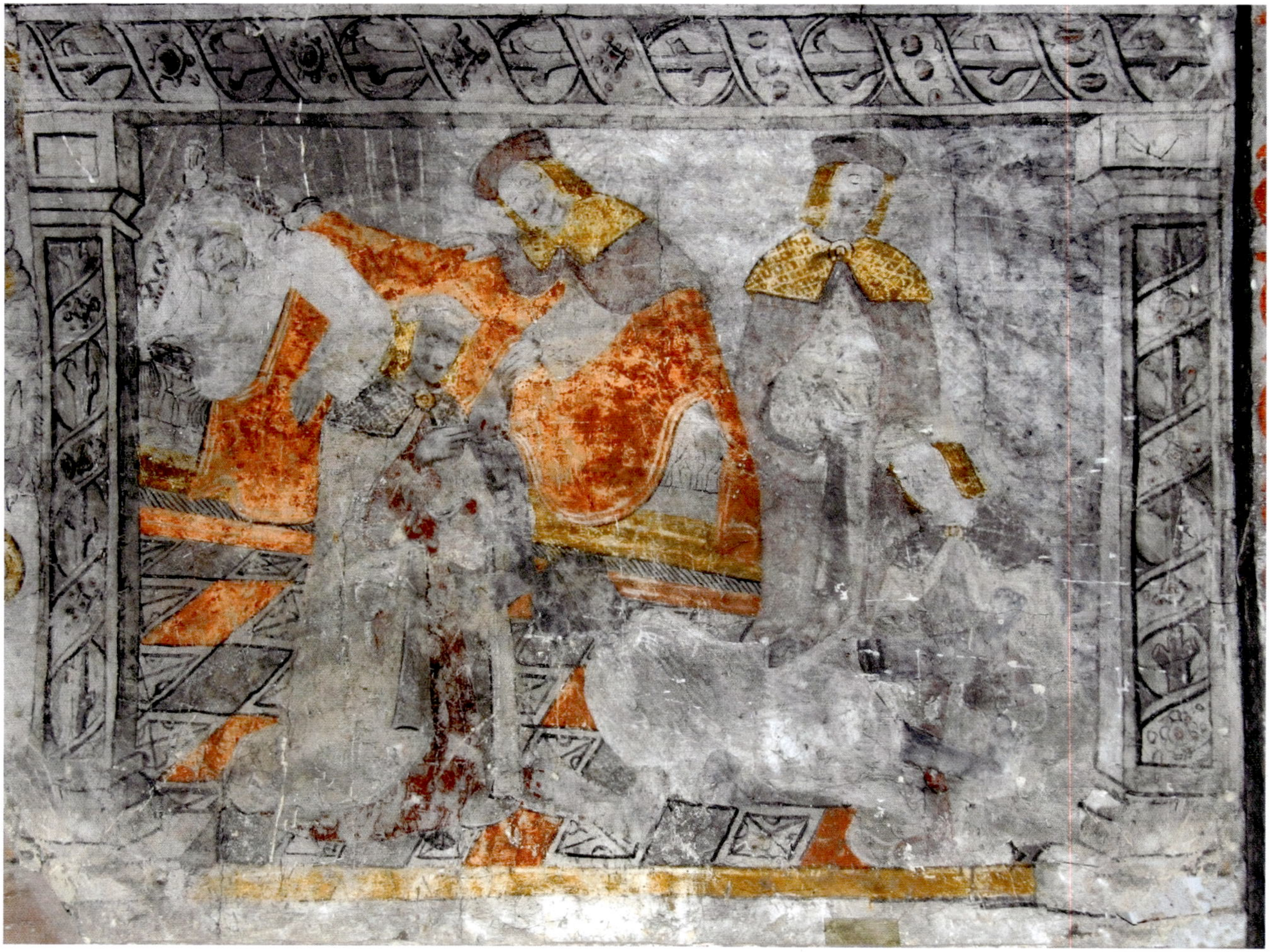

23. **Anonymous,** *fresco,* 15th century. Iglesia Parroquial, Basconcillos del Tozo (Spain).

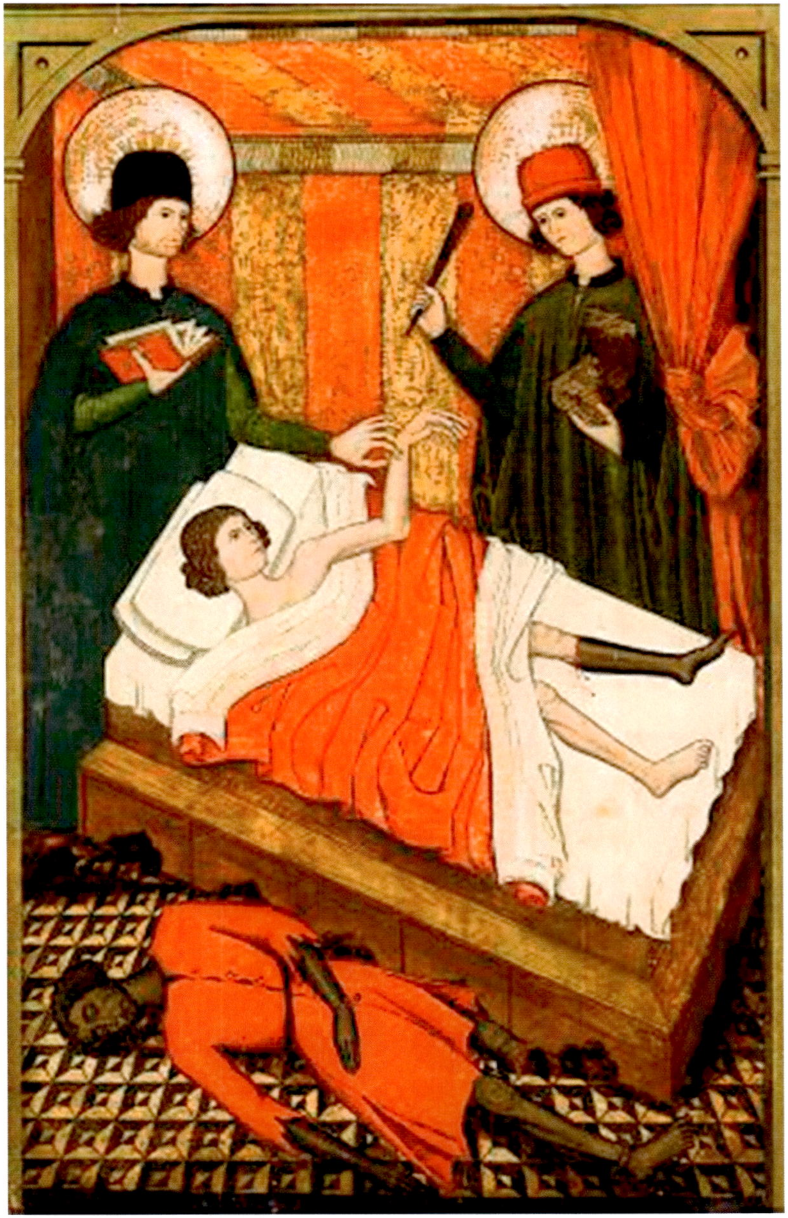

24. **unknown,** *panel,* 15th century? Private collection (Spain).

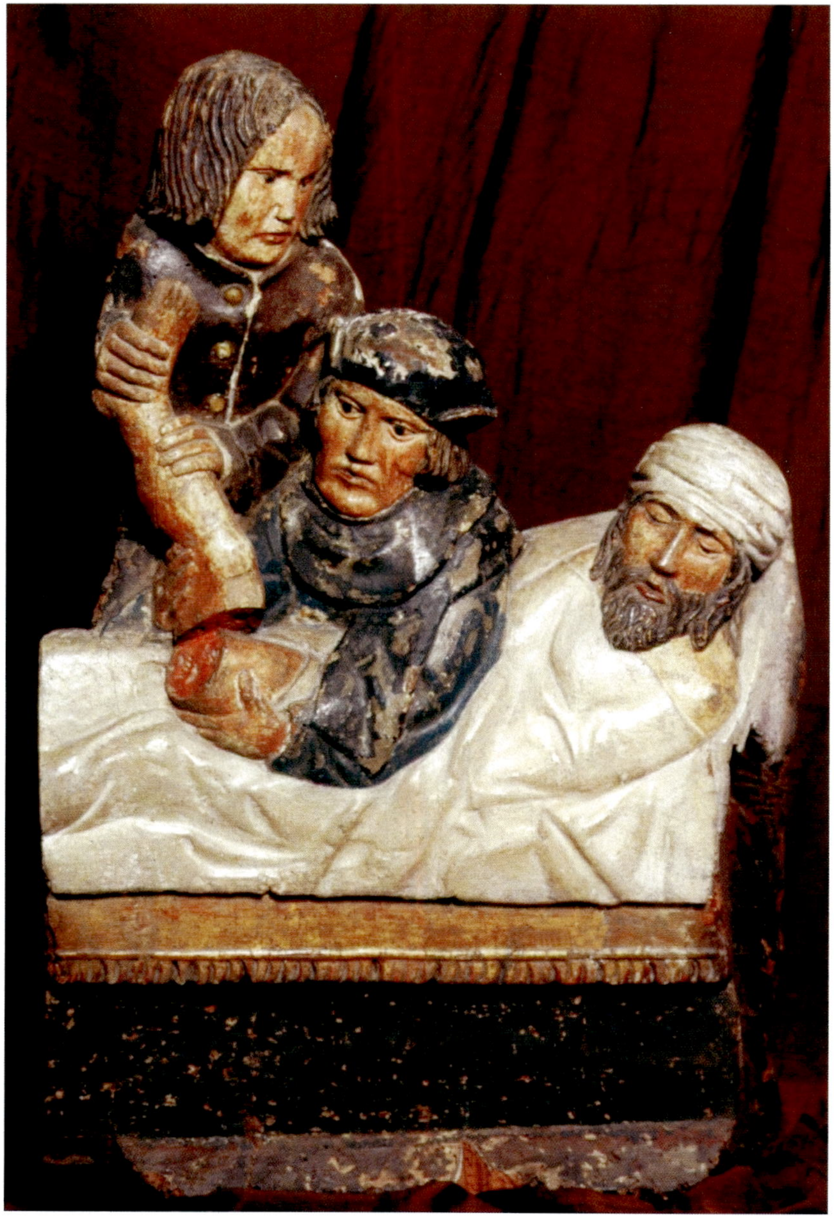

25. **Anonymous,** *woodcarving,* 15th century. Museum des Medizinhistorischen Instituts der Universität, Bern (Switzerland).

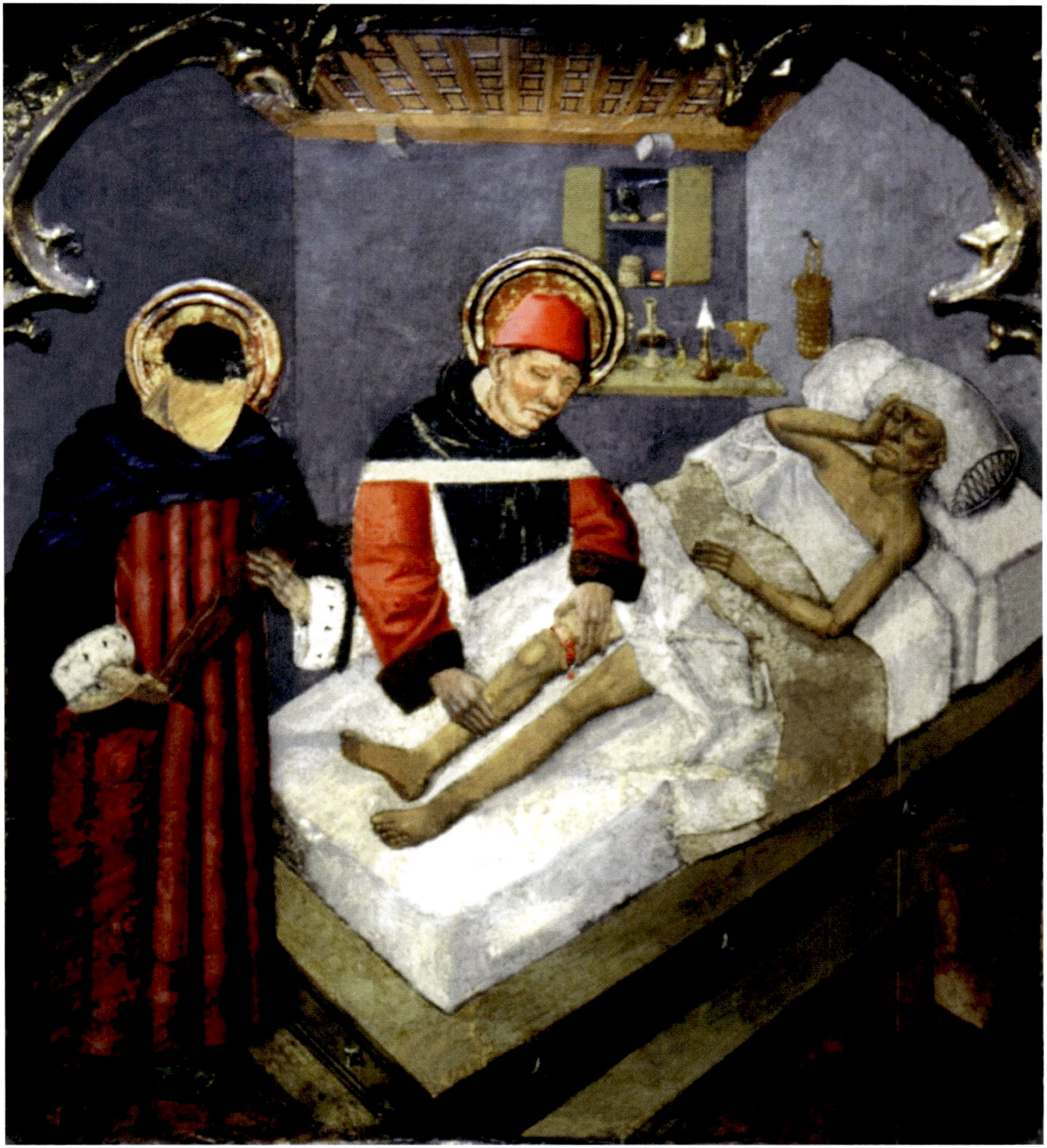

26. **Anonymous,** *panel of altarpiece,* 15th century. Retable de St. Jean l'évangéliste, L'église Sainte-Marie, Palau del Vidre (France).

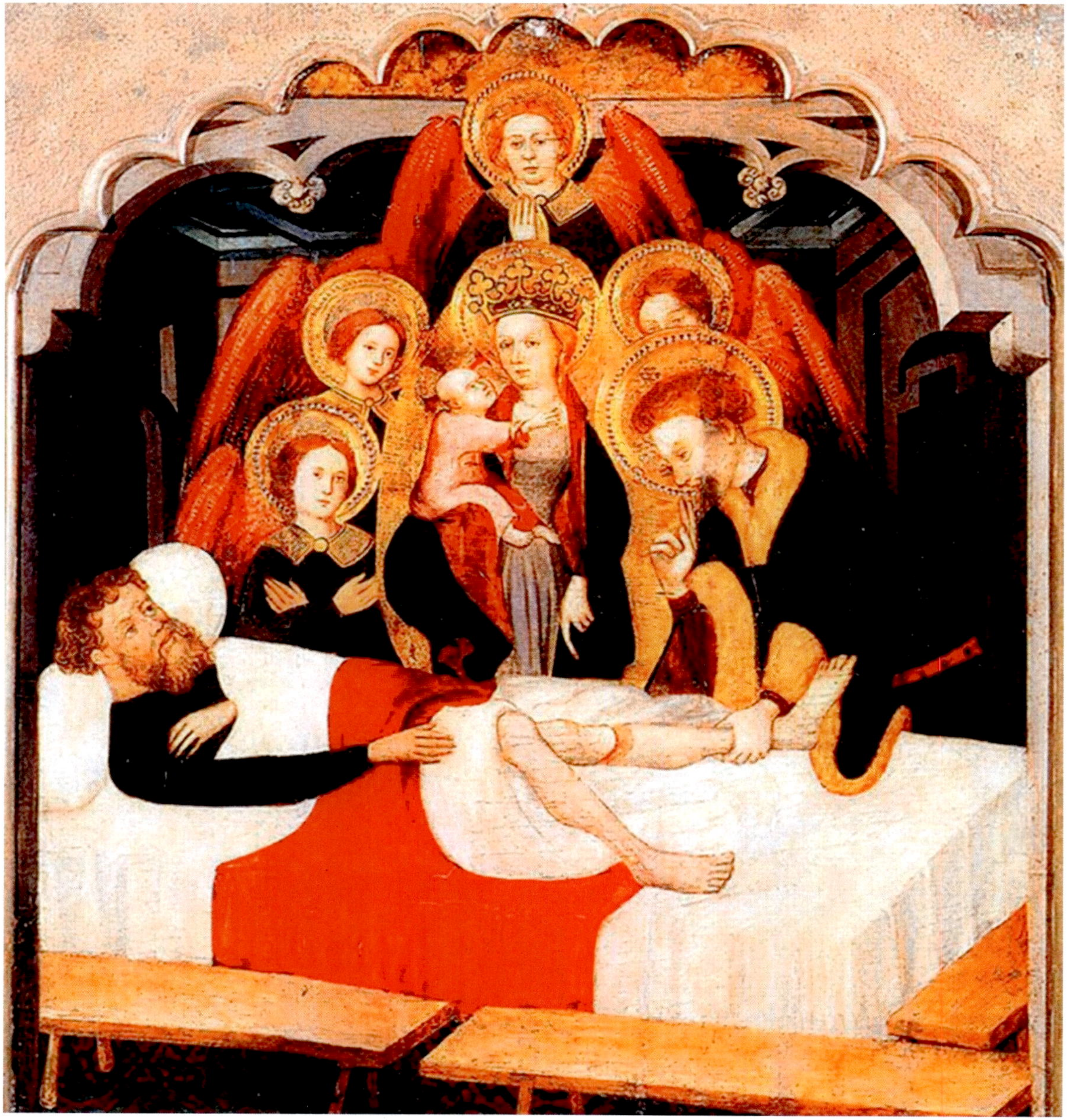

27. **Pupil of Luis Borrassá,** *panel,* 15th century. Museo Nacional del Prado 'Derechos reservados © Museo del Prado – Madrid, Madrid (Spain).

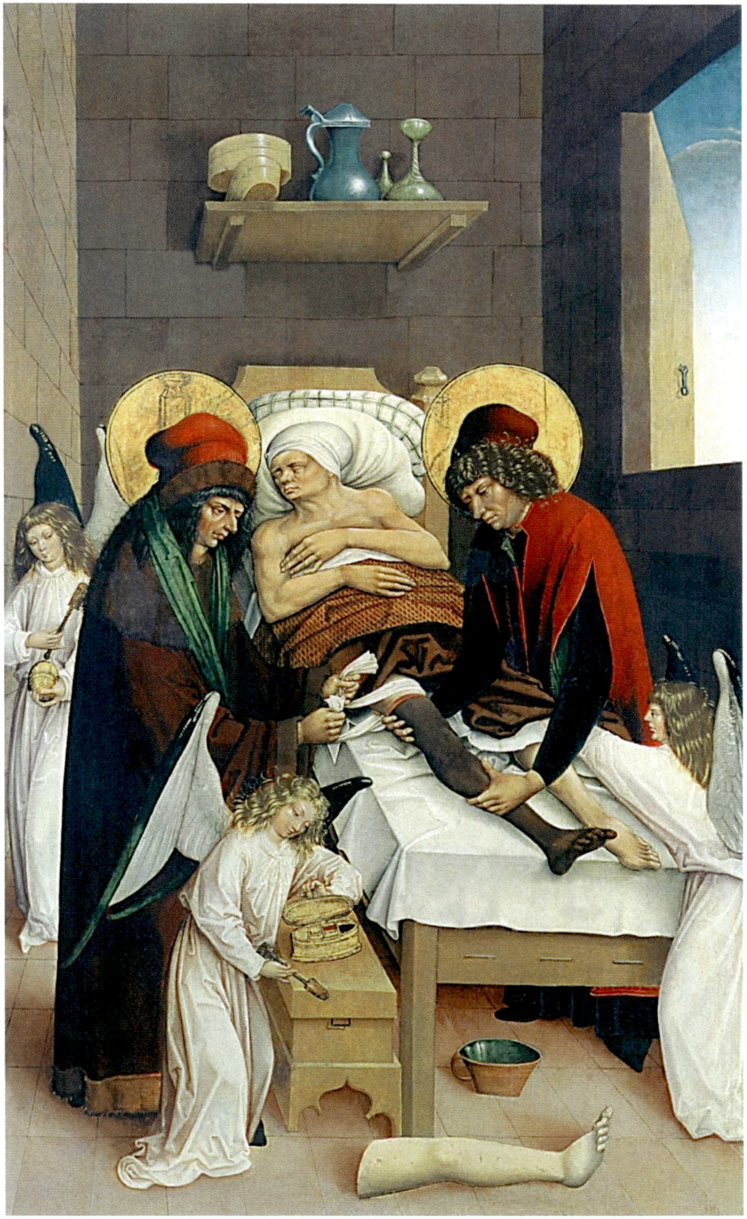

28. Anonymous, *painting*, end 15th -early16th century. Württembergisches Landesmuseum, Stuttgart (Germany).

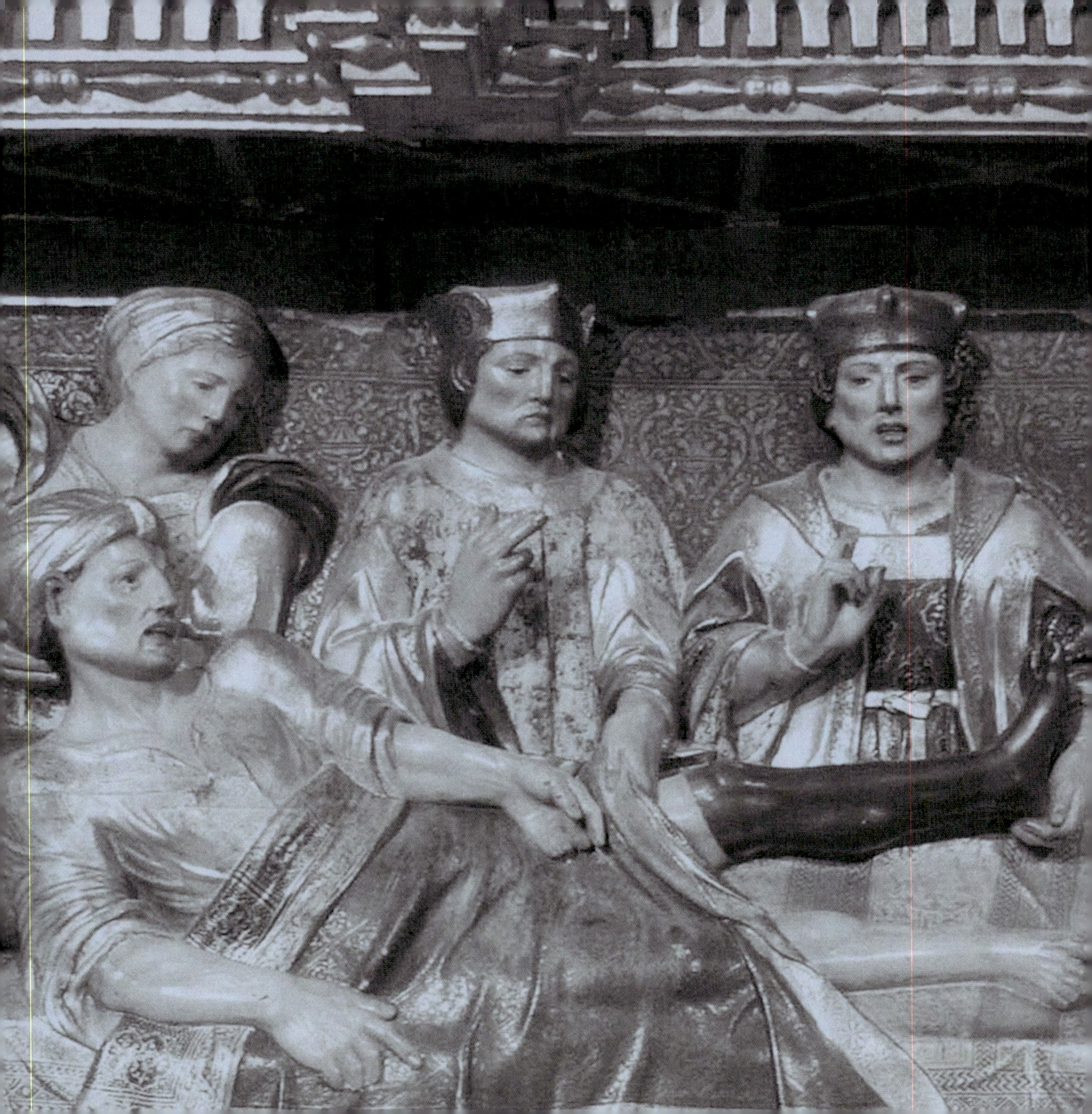

Spanish depictions of the Miracle of the Black Leg

Carmen Fracchia

The cult of Sts Cosmas and Damian was completely established in Spain by the seventh century. However, it was especially after the reconquest of Andalusia from the Moors in 1248 that churches dedicated to these holy doctors in urban centres such as Burgos, Leon, Oviedo, and Valencia spread throughout Spain.

The devotion of Cosmas and Damian in the crowns of Castile and Aragon was partly due to the presence of their relics. The acquisition of relics was essential for the creation of pilgrimage centres, the encouragement of the devotion of saints and the spread of the iconography of saints and their miracles in reliquaries either painted or carved. The circulation of images of Cosmas and Damian in Spain prepared viewers for the reception of the visual representation of the miraculous transplantation of the black leg from the end of the fourteenth century on. Devotion to Cosmas and Damian as well as representations of these saints were from the sixteenth century onwards also established in the Spanish colonies of the New World.

Medieval legends of healing saints, who perform miracles of body reparations, such as that of Cosmas and Damian, were written to counteract horror at the fragmentation of bodies which was performed in Western Europe for political or scientific purposes, between the end of the thirteenth century and the beginning of the following century. The legalization of dissection practices in European centres and the public exhibition of the body parts of criminals, associated with the judicial practice of torture, were the main causes. On the other hand, horror at the division of bodies of saints was lessened essentially because of their transformation into relics which fulfilled a didactic function. In the Christian imaginary, relics, contained and usually exhibited in caskets made of precious materials, signify the physical presences of saints.

Early representations of the Miracle of the Black Leg in Spain

The *Acta Sanctorum* recorded the presence of the relics of saints Cosmas and Damian in the year 972 in the Collegiate church dedicated to the martyr brothers in Covarrubias, south of the royal seat of Burgos. It is in this church that we find one of the first Spanish representations of the Miracle of the Black Leg (Ill. 19 page 68) in the crown of Castile. Dating from around 1496, it is by the Castilian painter

Pedro Berruguete. This scene is the only surviving panel of an altarpiece devoted to Cosmas and Damian commissioned by Abbot Diego Fernández de Castro, a relative of Pope Sixtus IV.

Berruguete executed the altarpiece of Cosmas and Damian after his return from Italy, where he must have become familiar with the first European representations of the Miracle of the Black Leg, codified by Tuscan artists in the late fourteenth century. In his version, however, Berruguete concentrates only on the episode of the grafting operation which becomes the focus of his composition. It is a bizarre image, in which only the verger's legs can be seen. The patient's upper body is hidden from view as he lies behind the holy doctor who is performing the transplantation of the black leg in the foreground of the image. The saint is in charge of the operation under the concentrated watch of three young witnesses, two women and a man, while his holy brother is looking at their patient.

The absence of the Ethiopian "organ-donor" from Berruguete's image is a reminder of the law promulgated by the Catholic Monarchs during the last decade of the fifteenth century ordering the expulsion of the Moors from the crowns of Castile and Leon. The Ethiopian is also absent in the contemporary version of this miracle painted by the Master of the Balbases, who has been identified with the wealthy trader-painter Andrés Sánchez de Oña (Ill. 22 page 71). In his panel, which was originally in the royal church of Cosmas and Damian in Burgos, Sánchez de Oña replaces Berruguete's witnesses by three angels. They form a Hispano-Flemish visual motif that emphasizes the medieval folkloric theme of the loss and restoration of body parts. The Castilian artist also decided to depict the verger's discarded wounded white leg, which is held by the angel on the right of the composition.

Andrés Sánchez de Oña and the painter Alonso de Sédano (who was previously identified as the Master of Los Balbases) were also in charge of the decoration of the reliquary of Cosmas and Damian in the Cathedral of Burgos.

The corpse of the Ethiopian is invisible in later versions of the transplantation of the black leg in Spain: in a painting on wood in Sitges, near Barcelona (Ill. 31 page 94) and in two relief panels from polychrome wood altarpieces. One is in Hontoria del Pinar, in the province of Burgos, executed by José Rodríguez, Mateo de Olmos and Pedro de Cicarte for the church dedicated to the holy doctors (Ill. 55 page 118). The other panel is in the church of St Peter in Teruel, in the kingdom of Aragon (Ill. 45 page 108), where the anonymous artist added, instead, the presence of three witnesses to this miracle, as Berruguete had previously done, following the Tuscan tradition.

The corpse of the Ethiopian donor in the Spanish tradition. The concept of the "Ethiopian" in early modern Spain

The invisibility of the Ethiopian's corpse is not however a common feature in the Spanish tradition. The image of the Ethiopian, in this specific iconography, occasionally and radically departs from De Voragine's legend of the Miracle of the Black Leg and the Tuscan visual code of this legend. Therefore, it is important to pause at this stage and consider the concept of the "Ethiopian" in early modern Spain: who was he and how was the visual representation of this subject perceived by his contemporaries?

In the social collective European and Christian imaginary, De Voragine's Ethiopian partakes of the interchangeability of the terms and notions of "African" and "black", which dates back to antiquity and the beginning of the Christian era. In imperial Spain, however, the word "black" (*negro*) or "African" most often signifies "slave", whether it be a black person from sub-Saharan Africa, a Berber from North Africa, or an Iberian Muslim, but not a white slave from Turkey.

Most black people were captured by the Spaniards, but particularly by the Portuguese, in Africa, in present-day Guinea-Bissau, Guinea Conakry, Senegal, Gambia, part of Mali, and part of Burkina. Slaves were then transported to Seville to be sold at auctions on the steps of the Cathedral or in the square of San Francisco, and from there they were exported to the rest of the peninsula, to important urban centres such as Burgos, Valladolid, Barcelona and Valencia, and also to the New World. In Spain, the price of a slave, which depended on the person's physical condition, age and sex, rose during the sixteenth century, at the height of the Iberian slave trade. In the cities, slaves, who were branded, were mainly employed in domestic service, which explains why black women usually attracted higher prices.

The creation of slave trade licences by the State, granted by the House of Trade and the Council of the Indies, established in Seville from the beginning of the sixteenth century, turned this business of trading human beings into an efficient and profitable system. At the peak of the slave trade at the end of the sixteenth century, Seville became the main slave market in the Spain, followed by Valencia. Seville had the largest slave community in the crowns of Castile and Aragon: its population of 120,000 included approximately 30,000 slaves black and white. There was also a high proportion in Madrid, the seat of the Habsburg Court from 1560. During the seventeenth century, however, the slave trade began to decline, owing to a series of events which contributed to the gradual decrease of the population. Decisive causes were the expulsion of over 30,000 *Moriscos* (Muslims converted to Christianity) in 1609-14, the loss of Portugal (under Spanish rule from 1581 to 1640), and the death of 46% of the population during the plague of 1640.

The prominent presence of black people in urban Spain and especially in Seville led contemporary commentators to compare the city to a "giant chessboard containing an equal number of white and black chessmen".

The monopoly of the slave trade since the fifteenth century and the subsequent highest concentration of African slaves in Spain created specific social conditions such as the clear demarcation between slaves and servants and the foundation of exclusively "black" confraternities in urban centres in the crowns of Castile and Aragon.

The African presence during the fifteenth and sixteenth centuries in Iberia was higher than in the rest of Western Europe. Given these conditions, it is remarkable that the Spanish visual representation of black slaves is rare compared to its Western European counterpart. It is well known that the presence of Africans in Early Modern Europe was rendered visible through religious subjects, of which the most popular was the *Adoration of the Magi*. It was first introduced to Spain *c.* 1470 by Hans Memling, in the central panel of the *Adoration of the Magi* triptych (Prado Museum, Madrid), displayed on the altar of Charles V's chapel in the castle of Aceca, near Aranjuez. In Spain, this imagery coexists with another religious depiction, the Miracle of the Black Leg. In contrast, images of chained Afro-Hispanic slaves were only codified in the sixteenth century by European artists born outside Spain: this iconography had no resonance in Spanish art.

The documentation available on different aspects of the slave trade in the crowns of Castile and Aragon establishes that blackness had become a mark of a social condition or else a signifier of lack of freedom. The range of arbitrary and contradictory colour classifications included in the word "black" meant that it inevitably gave rise to the impression that any black person was a slave. This is clearly the context in which early modern Spanish viewers approach the representations of the Miracle of the Black Leg.

Depiction of the non-European donor

It is interesting to note the position that the corpse of the Ethiopian, occupies in the composition of the image of the Spanish Miracle of the Black Leg when it is faithful to De Voragine's tale and to the Tuscan visual prototype. This is the interpretation adopted by the painter and sculptor León Picardo, who worked for powerful political and ecclesiastical clients such as the Grand Inquisitor and Regent Francisco Jiménez de Cisneros, known as the "missionary of the Moors".

Picardo's painting was made for an altarpiece at the Cathedral of Burgos (Ill. 35 page 98), home of the relics of Cosmas and Damian. The reliquary was decorated by Andrés Sánchez de Oña, another painter of the Miracle of the Black Leg. In Picardo's image, the painter shows the transplantation of the black leg in the foreground with no further anecdotal distractions. The open window of the sacristy leads to the background showing the cemetery of the church of St Peter-in-Chains. We can clearly see that one of the holy doctors is lifting the shroud from the Ethiopian's corpse while his twin brother cuts off one of the cadaver's legs to be grafted on to the white verger's body.

A similar amputation scene is also visible in the background of the predella scene by Jaume Huguet. He was the most prestigious artist in Barcelona in the middle of the fifteenth century, where he worked for confraternities and collaborated with the painter Miquel Nadal who depicted a different version of this theme, as we shall see later.

Huguet's image of the Miracle of the Black Leg for the church of Santa María de Terrasa, near Barcelona, was carried out in 1460 for an altarpiece dedicated to the saints Abdon and Sennen, royal martyrs from Persia under Roman persecution (Ill. 15 page 64). The cult of Abdon and Sennen was very popular in the crown of Aragon as was the cult of Cosmas and Damian who were also of eastern origin and victims of the Roman Empire.

Huguet depicts the royal Persian couple in the central panel of his altarpiece. He places the image of Cosmas and Damian, the scenes depicting their martyrdom and their Miracle of the Black Leg in the predella.

In an anonymous fifteenth-century fresco, which is in a very poor condition, in the parish church of Basconcillos del Tozo, in the province of Burgos, the holy doctors appear twice: in the background with the patient and in the foreground with the donor (Ill. 23 page 72). The artist unusually shifts the scene of the mutilation of the Ethiopian, where a fragment of his leg to be amputated is visible, closer to the viewer. This is an important detail since after 1492 the shift of the mutilated African corpse to the foreground of the composition becomes more prominent. This is not surprising if we consider the political impact that the last decade of the fifteenth century had on the building of the Spanish empire: the expulsion of all Jews from the crowns of Castile and Aragon, the Reconquest of Granada – which was the last Muslim stronghold in the Iberian Peninsula – and the discovery of the New World.

The version of the Miracle of the Black Leg (Ill. 21 page 70) by the Castilian court portraitist Fernando del Rincón de Figueroa for the Monastery of St Francis in Guadalajara testifies to the political significance of this period. The image of the mutilated Ethiopian corpse, wrapped in a shroud with the gangrenous white leg attached and with his face towards the spectator-believer, is placed on the floor parallel to the seated verger. Unusually, the artist has included another bizarre visual motif at the bottom right corner of the composition that shows one of three miracles worked by the holy doctors. It is a man who voids through his mouth a snake which had entered his body when he was asleep. This rare motif is erased in a contemporary copy made after Rincón de Figueroa (Ill. 43 page 106) which testifies to the popularity of this composition.

In his painting Rincón, court painter to Ferdinand the Catholic and the Emperor Charles V, introduces the interesting visual motif of the pomegranate on the central shelf behind the holy doctor in charge of the transplantation of the black leg on the right of the composition. This exotic fruit is the heraldic emblem of the city of Granada and evokes the final Reconquest of the Muslim city in 1492. The artist thus establishes a link between the legend of Cosmas and Damian and the Christianization of the infidels of Granada.

The pomegranate will be also shown a century later in a large representation of the Miracle of the Black Leg painted for the Carmelite Monastery of the Mártires in Granada (Ill. 41 page 104) by the painter and gilder Pedro de Raxis the Elder. It is placed on the verger's bed, in the foreground. This is a copy, signed in 1592, and made by the artist himself after his own painting of the Miracle of the Black Leg, which is no longer extant.

In his later interpretation, the Ethiopian donor is placed in the foreground of the image. However, he is not depicted as a corpse, but he is alive and sleeping, or perhaps sedated, lying naked on the floor with his head resting on a cushion by the verger's bed. In addition, Raxis depicts the exceptional transplantation of the white gangrenous leg, now miraculously healed, to the African body. This manner of representation is significant because the mutilated Ethiopian makes visible the possibility of the restoration and resurrection of his intact body.

The illusion of the realism of the Ethiopian body by Raxis, which is no longer covered by a shroud, departs from the representation of the African corpse of De Voragine's legend. Instead, the naturalistic treatment of the Ethiopian at rest on the floor constitutes one of the first portraits of an African slave in early modern Spain.

Raxis belonged to a dynasty of artists in Granada and was the head of an important artistic workshop there. He was in charge of prestigious decorative schemes such as those for the Hospital de Santiago in Úbeda, in Andalucía, founded by Diego de los Cobos, the Inquisitor and powerful bishop of Jaén. This experience gave Raxis direct contact with the poor, the sick and the dying. Early modern Spanish hospitals were formed out of the unification of medieval hospitals during the fifteenth century in the crown of Aragon and from the end of the following century in the crown of Castile. These institutions provided medical and social assistance to the poor, slaves amongst them. They were the result of Counter-Reformation thought which integrated the practice of charitable deeds into the discourses of the Catholic faith and salvation.

Raxis's motif of the sedated Ethiopian with his anointed and healed white leg also occurs in a seventeenth-century panel of the Miracle of the Black Leg (Ill. 56 page 119) painted by an anonymous artist in the Santuario de Santa Eulalia de Mérida in Totana (today in the province of Murcia).

This specific iconography was also exported to New Spain (modern Mexico), where the cult of Sts Cosmas and Damian was established in the first half of the sixteenth century. They were the patrons of the Hospital del Buen Amor de Dios, founded by the Franciscan friar Juan de Zumárraga in Mexico City, capital of the Viceroyalty of New Spain, in 1547. He was the first bishop, archbishop and Inquisitor of New Spain, and oversaw the building of the metropolitan Cathedral. Here in 1666, in the chapel dedicated to Cosmas and Damian, appears a depiction of the Miracle of the Black Leg (Ill. 52 page 115). This episode takes place in the portico of a colonial hospital with a view of a small fountain set against the wall of an exotic wooded area on the left of the composition. The sedated Ethiopian with the gangrenous white leg attached to his body is resting on a pillow on a typical woven mat. He looks at the viewer, with a cat in the foreground. This anecdotal tone is complemented by the representation of Cosmas and Damian as contemporary Mexican physicians, graduates of the Real y Pontificia Universidad de México (Royal and Pontifical University of Mexico), with their long black academic gowns and short golden capes. To emphasize the physical reality of the miracle, the artist has also added a contemporary bow-saw, which has just been used in the amputation process. It is partially hidden between the bed post and the Ethiopian's left leg. This exquisite painting is a predella scene for the altarpiece devoted to the twin martyrs by Mexican painter Sebastián López Dávalos. In the same year when he depicted the Miracle of the Black Leg, he was also one of the artists in charge of the first inspection of the miraculous image of Our Lady of Guadalupe, patron of Mexico.

A radical departure from De Voragine's legend

The visual motif of the attached gangrenous white leg to the Ethiopian body, even if this is not a miraculous transplantation, signifies the inclusion of Africans in the Christian discourse of the salvation of slaves. In the Spanish empire, the unconditional dependence of slaves on their masters was fundamental. The interaction of slavery and Christianity influenced the production of a small group of Castilian images of the Miracle of the Black Leg in the first half of the sixteenth century, at the peak of the early modern Spanish transatlantic slave trade. In this specific group of images, the transplantation of the gangrenous white leg to the Ethiopian donor is completely eliminated. However, the most striking departure from De Voragine's legend is the image of the living and mutilated African man in agony. This disturbing new visual motif of the Ethiopian in the Castilian Miracle of Sts Cosmas and Damian radically departs from the European iconography of the transplantation of the black leg. The mutilated Ethiopian is no longer depicted as a corpse or as a sedated man. He has been replaced by a mutilated living African man in the foreground of the composition, closer to the believer, and would have been perceived as the portrayal of a contemporary slave.

The earliest image of this extraordinary tradition from the crown of Castile is a bas-relief panel on the small altarpiece in polychrome wood dedicated to Cosmas and Damian in the chapel of St Gregory in the Cathedral of Palencia (Ill. 34 page 97). It was executed by the famous architect and sculptor Felipe Vigarny. He worked together with other painters of this miracle, Picardo and Berrugete's son Alonso, in Burgos Cathedral. Vigarny also shared their prestigious and influential clients, such as Cardinal Inquisitor Cisneros.

The St Gregory chapel belonged to the powerful Dominican friar Alonso de Burgos, confessor of the Catholic Monarchs. He was also appointed President of the Royal Council of Castile, which sponsored Columbus's voyages of discovery to the Indies. Alonso de Burgos's nephew, Juan de Arce, is buried in this chapel. Arce commissioned the altarpiece devoted to Cosmas and Damian from Vigarny. The artist placed his client in the large predella scene of the Miracle of the Black Leg, kneeling in prayer on the left between St John the Baptist and the head of the bed where the verger lies.

All personages, with the exception of the Ethiopian, are concentrated on the miraculous transplantation of his black leg: in the centre of the composition, the white verger is awake, and a young woman supports his head and stands behind the bed facing the viewer next to the holy doctors who are blessing their patient. On the left of the panel are Juan de Arce, who represents the viewer, and St John the Baptist; on the right is a man who is supposed to be Vigarny's self-portrait. He supports the verger's gangrenous leg and stands behind the living Ethiopian, who is fainting from the pain. Although the African donor does not occupy the centre of this composition, the realism and the naturalism of the representation of his body in agony are highlighted against the sumptuous gilding and transformed into an image of a contemporary slave. Thus, the living Ethiopian paradoxically becomes the centre of attention for the viewer, who cannot ignore his presence, unlike Cosmas and Damian and their witnesses to the transplantation of the black leg.

The realism of the Miracle of the Black Leg in a polychrome wood bas-relief panel on an altarpiece in Valladolid (Ill. 38 page 101) is stronger than that of Vigarny's predella in Palencia. The Valladolid panel, perhaps intended for a small confraternity in this imperial city, is attributed to the Castilian sculptor Isidro Villoldo. It is dated either 1539 or 1547. Villoldo, who was a key artist in sixteenth-century Toledo, Ávila and Seville, worked with Vigarny in the Cathedral of Toledo after the latter completed the Palencia panel.

Villoldo's realism highlights the expression of pain in the face of the living African man who is holding his mutilated left leg in his right hand. Unusually, the chopping block where the amputation of his leg took place is depicted below his stump. The chopping block was an essential tool used by surgeons to save the lives of wounded men on contemporary Spanish battlefields.

Indeed, in rural and urban centres in Spain surgeons were held by the regulations of the confraternities of Sts Cosmas and Damian. From 1501 onwards, surgeons had to provide certificates of purity of blood stating that they were without "Moorish, Jewish or African blood". Most anatomized bodies in these medical institutions came from the poor and the executed. Dissections of bodies of the executed were allowed in the medical "confraternities" There is evidence of this practice from the fourteenth century in the crown of Aragon and from the fourth decade of the sixteenth century in the crown of Castile. It is significant that images of the Miracle of the Black Leg were codified in the wealthiest Spanish slave cities, which also had universities for the study of anatomy.

Villoldo had previously been responsible for the design of the Miracle of the Black Leg in a relief in the choir stalls in the Cathedral of Ávila (Ill. 30 page 93). This work was started in 1534 by sculptors Lucas Giraldo and Juan Rodríguez and completed a decade later by Nicolás Cornielis de Holanda.

Villoldo's composition in Ávila is echoed in his small bas-relief in Valladolid. In the latter the polychrome but predominantly gilded wood of the panel highlights the incongruity of the mutilation of the elegant living African man, who would have been perceived as a contemporary slave.

It is important to add that slaves were not only commodities, but also fulfilled the function of being an ornament to their masters and an enhancement of their social status. The treatment of domestic slaves depended on the owner's economic and social position. However, it is important to notice that there was a fundamental difference between a domestic slave and a servant. While both were at the bottom of the social scale in terms of marginalization and exploitation, their means of reproduction and therefore of survival were different, as the servant was never auctioned or captured in wars. In some cases, the rigid domestic hierarchy in the Spanish household did not exclude an ambiguity in the relationship between slave and master, and in fact some slaves also achieved a closer relationship with their owners.

The new Castilian interpretation of De Voragine's tale will be reproduced, a century later, in the Miracle of the Black Leg (Ill. 51 page 114) by an anonymous painter for an altarpiece dedicated to Cosmas and Damian. Tiberio Damián, an Italian surgeon from the Hospital of San Hermenegildo in Seville, donated this painting in 1657 to the Jesuit Church of the Annunciation in the same city (today known as the University Chapel). The unknown artist also introduced two new details into this interpretation. These are the presence of surgical tools in the foreground of a hospital room and the unusual depiction of the white verger in agony. His amputated leg is tied with a tourniquet and he is neither asleep nor sedated, calm or surprised; he is awake and in agony. Instead of the traditional Spanish or European depiction of a calm verger, showing no pain, this patient is shown as being restrained by one of the holy doctors and two assistants, while the other surgeon saint performs the transplantation of the black leg.

This group of Castilian paintings is faithful to only one key element of the Latin legend of the Miracle of the Black Leg: the indifference shown by Cosmas and Damian and the white verger towards the Ethiopian. This attitude is more evident in the images where the African corpse becomes the mutilated and living Ethiopian who reclines on the floor, closer to the believer. These Castilian visual forms seem to display a knowledge of the means of control applied to the social behaviour of the slave population by "local police forces", known as the Holy Brotherhood (*Santa Hermandad*). One of its responsibilities was the regulation of crime and there are records of punishment practices against slaves, such as the amputation of ears, hands and feet. These practices might have been quite regular, given the constant preoccupation expressed by Spanish theologians and intellectuals. They gave instructions to slave owners on how to treat their slaves and the ways in which they should avoid the death of their slaves, so that they could maximize their investment and profits.

Representations of the Miracle inspired by the Greek legend of Sts Cosmas and Damian

The religious image of the transplantation of the black leg in Spain, and in particular in the crown of Castile, symbolizes the violence of slavery in imperial Spain. This is more obvious when we turn our attention to another group of images depicting the Miracle of Sts Cosmas and Damian produced mainly in the crown of Aragon. These images are not informed by De Voragine's tale. They probably followed the Greek legend of Cosmas and Damian, the oldest known version, written in the fifth century.

In the Greek source for the "Miracle of the holy and glorious *anargyri* (i.e. 'they who decline silver') Cosmas and Damian", the ethnicity of the healthy donor is not specified. One is led to assume that both the recipient and the donor of the leg belong to the same ethnic group. The location where the miraculous healing takes place is the church of St Theodosios the Cenobiarch (423-590), who was from Cappadocia (modern Turkey). The time of death of the donor is specified as a period of "four days". The Greek literary source, which is a more anecdotal text than De Voragine's, is peppered with dialogues emphasizing the nature and practice of magical healing, the relevance of prayers and the vital role of the intercession of saints to inspire devotion: "They [Sts Cosmas and Damian] said to him [their patient after the operation], 'Go, brother. The mighty works of God have been accomplished because your faith has saved you.'"

The Greek legend seems to inspire the panel of the Miracle of Sts Cosmas and Damian in the Cathedral of Barcelona (Ill. 14 page 63) by the painter Miquel Nadal. The miraculous leg is not black but white and the donor is not depicted. This complex image was painted for the altarpiece of the chapel of Cosmas and Damian commissioned by the ecclesiastic Francisco Desplá from Bernardo Martorell the Younger and Nadal, who completed the work by 1454.

Nadal introduces another unusual visual motif into the Spanish depictions of this subject: the image of a sitting man sleeping by the verger's bed in the foreground of the composition. It shows the artist's knowledge of the Italian device deployed in these depictions since the fourteenth century to signify that the miracle of the transplantation of the healthy leg took place at night.

Nadal also added two angels as assistants to the holy doctors; his colleague Huguet (Ill. 15 page 64) adopts them in his version, which follows De Voragine's Latin tale. Both compositions show the uncommon detail of the man's cancerous leg, with bleeding wounds dripping on to the floor as if the amputated leg still belongs to the verger's body; the leg is displayed beside by the verger's bed in Nadal's panel and on top of it in Huguet's predella, in the foreground, on the right of their images. This unusual visual motif indicates that both artists were also familiar with another literary source of the transplantation of the black leg. This description of the patient's cancerous leg is only found in the earliest Catalan legend of the Miracle of the Black Leg, written in the fifteenth century: "the spreading sore on the man's leg". This legend, "Miracle and exemplum of St Cosmas and St Damian of a young man who lost a leg through a malady of cancer, as recounted in the Lombardy Legend (i.e. *The Golden Legend*)", is considered to be among the seven earliest written versions of the legend of the miracle of the black leg that circulated in Europe.

The Greek version of the Miracle of Cosmas and Damian is also the literary source that inspires the Catalan panel painted by a pupil of the painter Luis Borrasá (Ill. 27 page 76). In this painting, executed in the first half of the fifteenth century, the absence of the Ethiopian and his black leg is evident. The patient is awake and calm and only one of the saints, possibly Cosmas, is depicted as a surgeon in charge of the grafting operation making a sign of blessing. Instead of his brother, the Virgin and Child surrounded by four angels occupy the centre of the composition, next to the holy doctor, to highlight the devotional tone of this miracle.

The black leg is also conspicuously absent from one of the seven terracotta roundels in relief (Ill. 29 page 92) made in 1504 for the monumental portal of the convent church of St Paula in Seville by Francisco Niculoso Pisano. The scene with the Miracle of the Black Leg portrays only the holy doctors and their patient who is awake and looking at the viewer, while one of the saints concentrates on the transplantation of a white leg. The donor of the healthy leg and the witnesses to the miraculous healing of the verger's body are also absent.

The black leg and the African donor are also absent from the twentieth-century version (Ill. 69 page 144) by painter E. Roja in the church of Santiago in the city of Lorca, now in the province of Murcia. The patient, who looks at the spectator, is at the centre of the composition. His saviours Cosmas and Damian stand at each side of his bed with their eyes towards the apparition of the Virgin and Child in the upper part of the composition. In this modern interpretation, there is only one visual detail of the miracle of the transplantation of the leg to be performed by the holy physicians. It is the small bleeding wound above the verger's right knee which the holy doctor on the right of the composition shows to the viewer. This visual motif indicates Roja's familiarity with the Greek source that specifies that the holy doctors "went and cut off the right leg of the dead man. They also cut off at the knee the right leg of the man who had the splinter and they placed the leg of the dead man against [the stump] of the [sick] man in the name of the Father, the Son, and the Holy Spirit. No sooner had they invoked the Holy Trinity than the man was found to be sound."

The Greek tale also explains why the holy doctors attached the discarded leg to their donor cadaver: "on the day of the resurrection, let each one take his own limb". The donor of the white leg, however, is absent from this group of Spanish images based on the Greek tale of Sts Cosmas and Damian.

Concluding remarks on the background of the Spanish interpretation of the Miracle of the Black Leg

The realism of the Castilian depiction of the living and mutilated Ethiopian and the contrast between the treatment of the body of the African donor and the European recipient transformed the original Tuscan visual depiction of the transplantation of the black leg. These innovations are symptomatic of slavery practices during the formation of the Spanish Empire. In the images produced in the slave cities of Ávila, Palencia, Valladolid, and Seville, the transplantation of the white leg to the African man is absent. In this respect, they echo the fourteenth-century depiction of De Voragine's tale in two paintings for the crown of Aragon: in the predella (Ill. 03 page 52) by Master of Rubió, perhaps the earliest image of the transplantation of the black leg in Spain, and in a panel now in a private collection (Ill. 24 page 73). While in the former painting the donor of the leg is a corpse, in the latter the anonymous painter depicts the sedated donor who lies down fully clothed on the floor and with no pain.

The Castilian images of the transplantation of the black leg, with the presence of the living mutilated African in the foreground of the composition and closer to the believer, focus on the violent appropriation of the donor's body and on his suffering. They also concentrate on the consequences of this action, the miraculous healing of the verger. This disturbing and violent visual motif in the Miracle of the Black Leg was a radical departure from the original Tuscan iconography. It also symbolizes the new phenomenon of *mestizaje* or ethnic intermixture between Spaniards, Native Americans and Africans in imperial Spain.

In these works, De Voragine's legend was manipulated by many factors: the discourses of exclusion and inclusion of African slaves in the social order; by the violence of slavery practices, where the relationship between slave owners and slaves was established by mercantile considerations; and also by the paradoxical correlation of protection and exploitation. In the sacred space of the pre-Counter-Reformation church, the sacrifice of the Ethiopian, who is perceived as a contemporary slave, in the visual form is justified by his total dependence and dedication to his master. This attitude seems to evoke the iconography of the wounded body of Christ and his generous sacrifice, death and resurrection to save humankind. The wounded body of the Christian martyr, such as Cosmas and Damian, is a central feature in Catholic Reformation Spain and in the discourses of salvation. The Castilian Miracle of the Black Leg codifies Christian discourse on slavery, which allows the violent inclusion of African slaves into the Spanish empire, and at the same time keeps them and their descendants at the margins of society.

Slavery was accepted as a natural phenomenon and as a constituent part of the social order by early modern Spanish intellectuals and theologians until the end of the nineteenth century. The causes and justification of slavery in imperial Spain are found in the Aristotelian doctrine of natural slavery, which was transformed in medieval times into a doctrine that justified the origin of slavery in the existence of sin and war. In the sixteenth century Spanish theologians followed the same lines of thought and agreed on the legitimization of slavery through war and heredity with the result that slavery was seen as a natural and indispensable component of life, necessary for domestic purposes. In fact, intellectuals such as Martín González de Cellorigo in his *Memorial de la política necesaria y* útil *restauración a la república de España y estados de ella* (*The Restoration of the Republic*), published in Valladolid in 1600, claimed that legal slavery was necessary because Spanish people were different by nature. However, some aspects of the system were questioned by the theologian and economist Tomás de Mercado in his *Suma de tratos y contratos* (*Manual of Deals and Contracts*), published in Seville in 1571. He declared that he was in favour of the slave market, but was in doubt regarding the legality of slaves captured without the justification of a just war. He also denounced the cruel treatment of slaves and pleaded for more humane behaviour from their masters.

The image of the transplantation of the black leg reinforced this complex attitude in the Spanish social imaginary. However, the new Castilian iconography of the living Ethiopian also opened up the possibility of depicting a new subject in high art: the contemporary African slave. His agony, pain or death paradoxically became the central focus of the viewer's attention. This religious image became a symbolic and folkloric vehicle for the depiction of contemporary Afro-Hispanic slaves in visual form before the iconographic measures devised by the Council of Trent were implemented in the crowns of Aragon and Castile.

The Spanish interpretation of the Miracle of the Black Leg was shaped by different factors that oscillated between the anxiety and terror of being recolonized by the "Moors" and the desire to keep under control ethnic intermixture at the peak of the Hispanic transatlantic slave trade.

In the Spanish colonies, the arrival of Africans from Spain and later from Africa contributed to the irreversibility of ethnic intermixture and the fear of fragmentation of imperial power. The traumatic phenomenon of slavery practices affected and manipulated the identity of the Ethiopian in the iconography of the Miracle of the Black Leg during the formation of the Spanish empire. These practices were shaped by the policies of expulsion of all Jews and Muslims from the crowns of Castile and Aragon, the constant fight against the Turks in the Mediterranean, and the discovery of new subjects and cultures in the New World.

Literature

Bugner, L., Devisse, J., Mollat M. (eds.). 1979. *The Image of the Black in Western Art*, vol. II, Lausanne.

David-Danel M.-L. 1958. *Iconographie des saints médecins Côme et Damien*, Lille.

Fracchia, C. 2007. 'Constructing the Black Slave in Spanish Golden Age Painting', in Nichols, T. (ed.). *Others and Outcasts in Early Modern Europe: Picturing the Social Margins*, Aldershot.

Fracchia, C. 2009. 'La problematización del blanqueamiento visual del cuerpo africano en la España Imperial y en Nueva España', *Revista Chilena de Antropología Visual*, 14, pp. 67-82.
Fracchia, C. 2010. 'El esclavo negroafricano en las imágenes españolas de los Santos Cosme y Damián', in Casares A. M. and Barranco M. G. (eds.), *La esclavitud negroafricana en la Historia de España. Siglos XVI y XVII*, Granada 127-49.
Gila Medina, L. 2003. 'Aproximación a la vida y obra del pintor y estofador alcalaíno-granadino Pedro Raxis', *Archivo Español de Arte*, 76, 389-406.
Gila Medina, L. 1987. 'Los Raxis: importante familia de artistas del Renacimiento Andaluz. A ella perteneció el gran escultor Pablo de Rojas', *Archivo Español de Arte*, 238, 167-77.
González, R.J. 1973. *Iconografía de los santos Cosme y Damián*, Barcelona.
López Campuzano, J. 1996. 'Iconografía de los Santos Sanadores (II): San Cosme y San Damián', *Anales de la Historia del Arte*, 6, 255-66.
Orozco Díaz, E. 1966. *Guía del Museo Provincial de Bellas Artes Granada. Palacio de Carlos V*, Madrid.
Parrado del Olmo, J.M. 1981. *Los escultores seguidores de Berruguete en Ávila*, Ávila.
Post, C.R. 1930-1966. *A History of Spanish Painting*, Cambridge.
Ruiz Gomar, R. 1993. 'Sebastián López Dávalos, Un pintor novohispano del siglo XVII', *Anales del Instituto de Investigaciones estéticas*, 16, 64, 15-29.
Silva Maroto, S., Pilar M. 2003. *Pedro de Berruguete: el primer pintor renacentista de la Corona de Castilla*, Valladolid.
Yarza Luaces, J. 2004. 'Algunas reflexiones sobre iconografía en Pedro Berruguete y su época', *Actas del Symposium Internacional Pedro Berruguete y su entorno. Palencia, 24-26 abril de 2003*, Palencia.

On early modern slavery in Imperial Spain:

Cortés Alonso, V. 1964. *La esclavitud en Valencia durante el reinado de los Reyes Católicos*, Valencia.
Cortés López, J.L. 1986. *Los orígenes de la esclavitud negra en España*, Salamanca.
Franco Silva, A. 1979. *La esclavitud en Sevilla y su tierra a fines de la Edad Media*, Sevilla.
Martín Casares, A. 2000. *La esclavitud en la Granada del siglo XVI: Género, raza y religión*, Granada.
Martín Casares, A., Barranco, M.G. (eds.). *La esclavitud negroafricana en la Historia de España. Siglos XVI y XVII*, Granada.
Vila Villar, E. 1977. *Hispanoamérica y el comercio de esclavos*, Sevilla.

On early modern Spanish history of surgery and medicine:

Granjel, L.S. 1968. *Cirugía española del Renacimiento*, Salamanca.
Granjel, L.S. 1980. *Historia general de la medicina española renacentista*, Salamanca.
López Piñero, J.M. 1976. *Medicina moderna y sociedad española. Siglos XVI – XX*, Valencia.

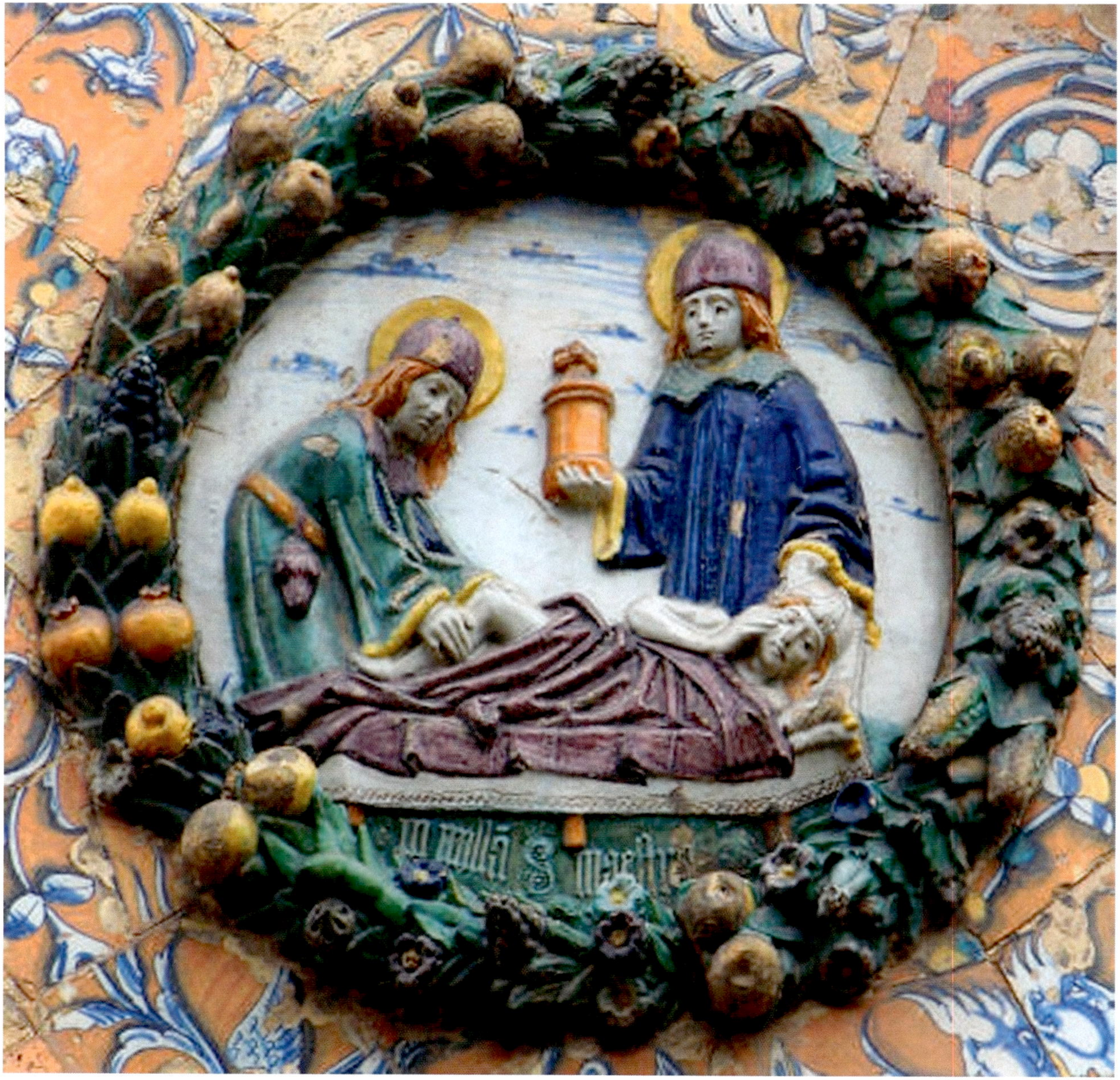

29. **Francisco Nicoloso Pisano,** (Pisa, ?- 1529, Sevilla), active 1498-ca. 1529, *terracotta roundel in relief,* 1504.
Monasterio de Santa Paula, Sevilla (Spain).

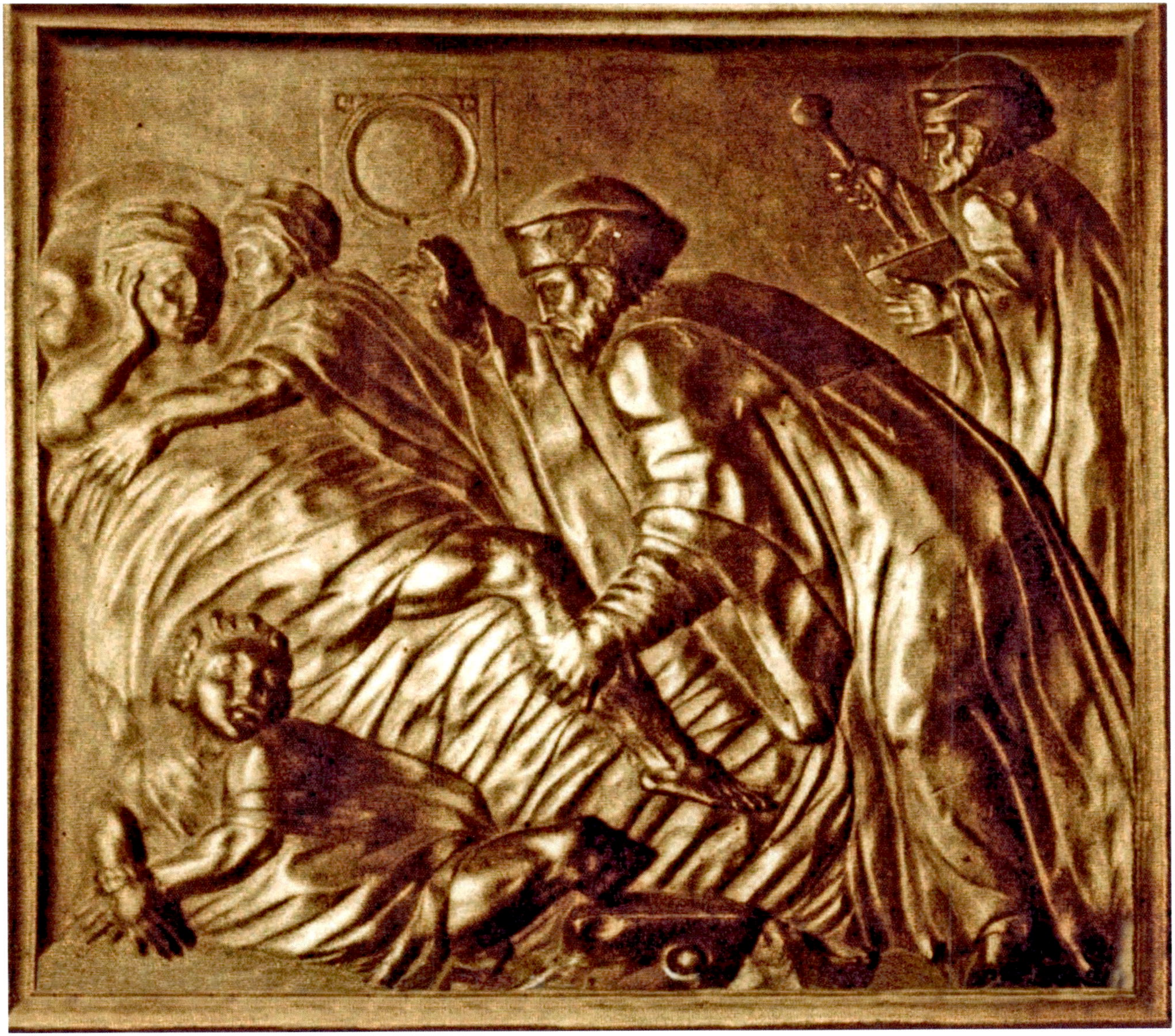

30. **Juan Rodriguez, Lucas de Giraldo, Nicolas Cornelis de Holanda,** *sculpture in wood (choir stall),* 1534-1544. Catedral, Ávila (Spain).

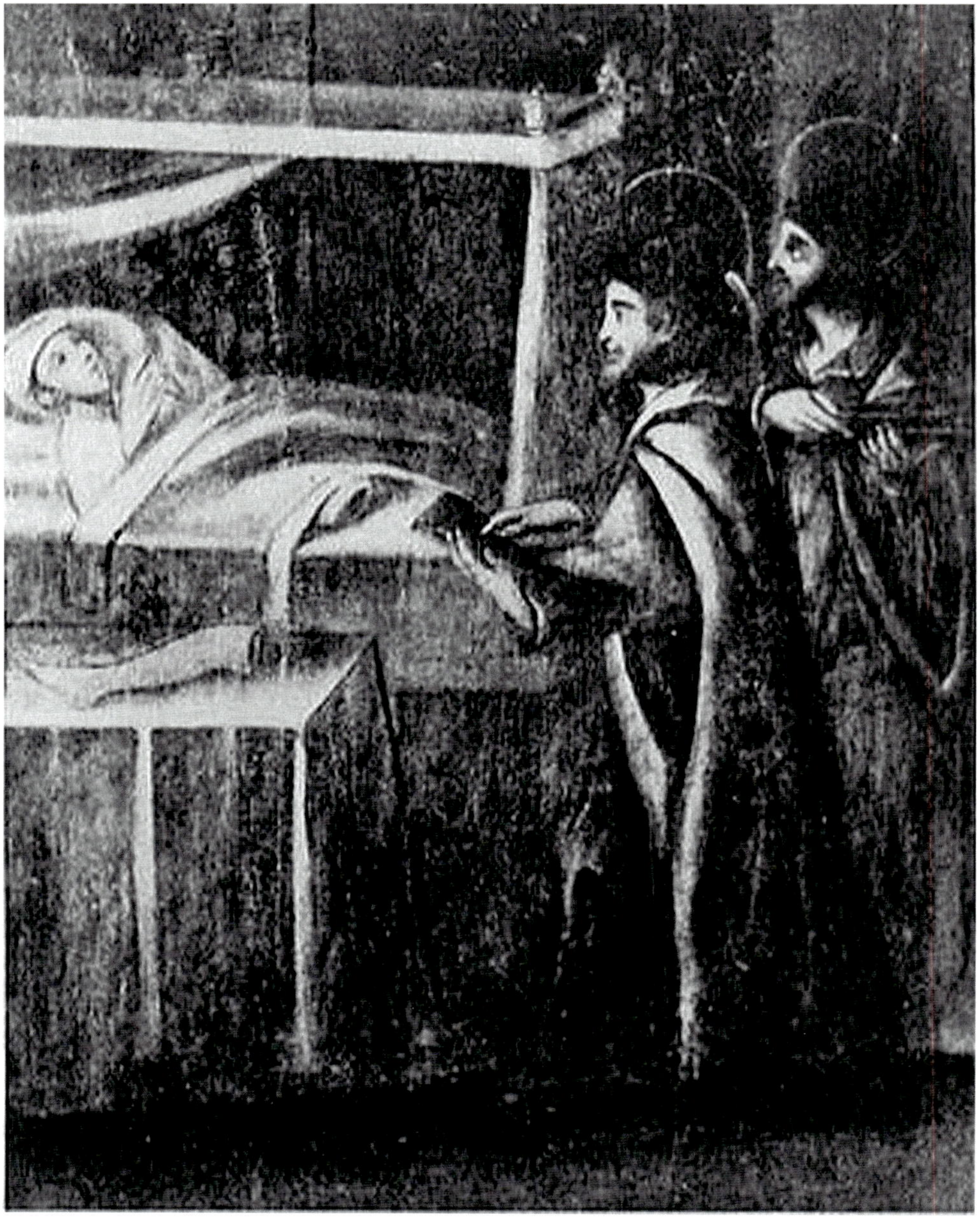

31. **unknown,** *panel?*, 16th century, whereabouts unknown (Spain? Formerly in the collection of Dr. Benaprés, Sitges, Spain).

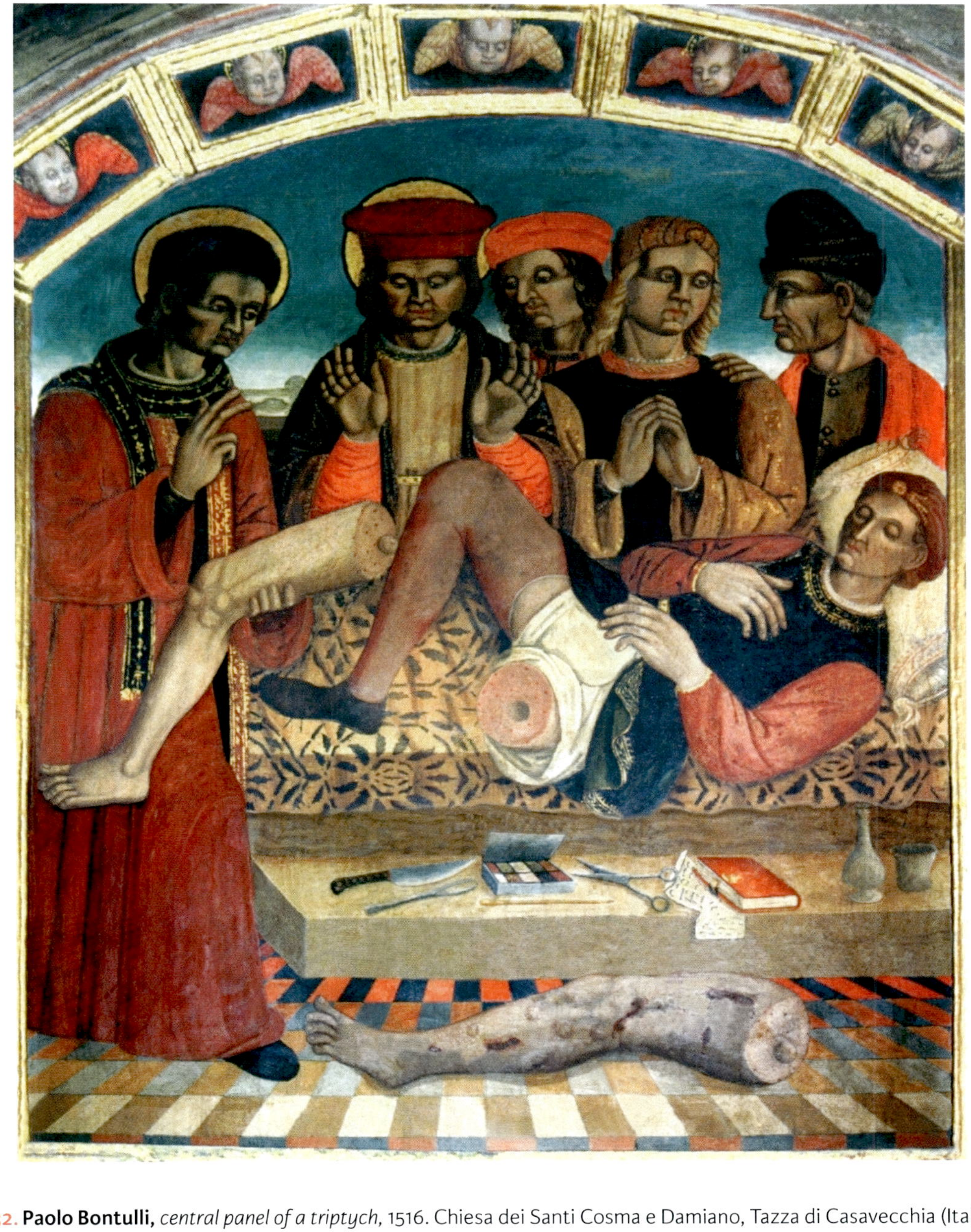

32. **Paolo Bontulli,** *central panel of a triptych,* 1516. Chiesa dei Santi Cosma e Damiano, Tazza di Casavecchia (Italy).

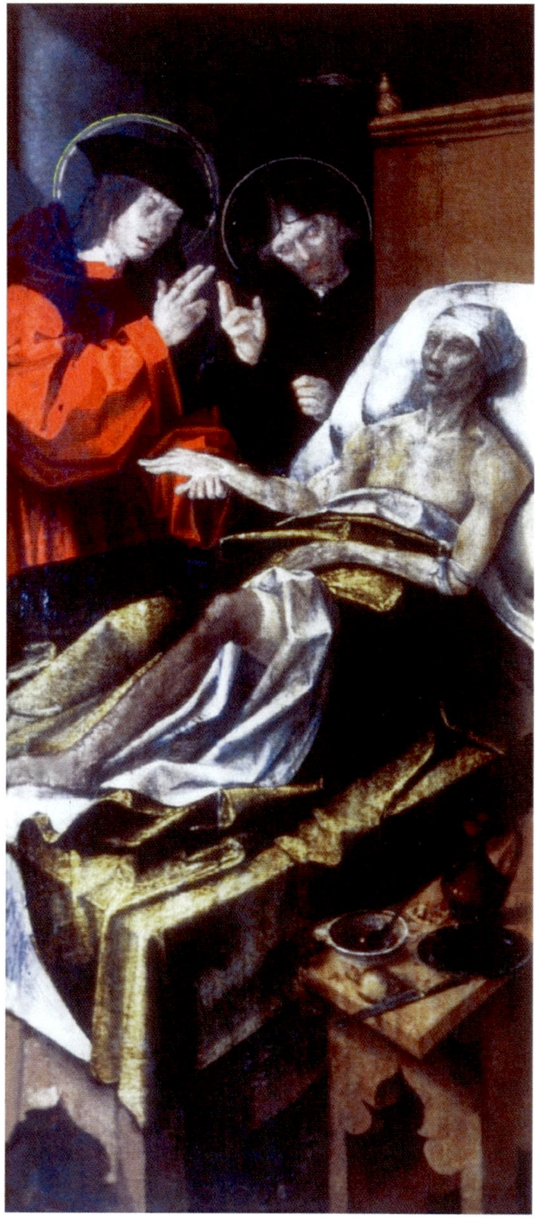

33. **Garcia Fernandes** (?-1565) *painting*, 1518-1540. Museo Machado do Castro, Coïmbra (Portugal).

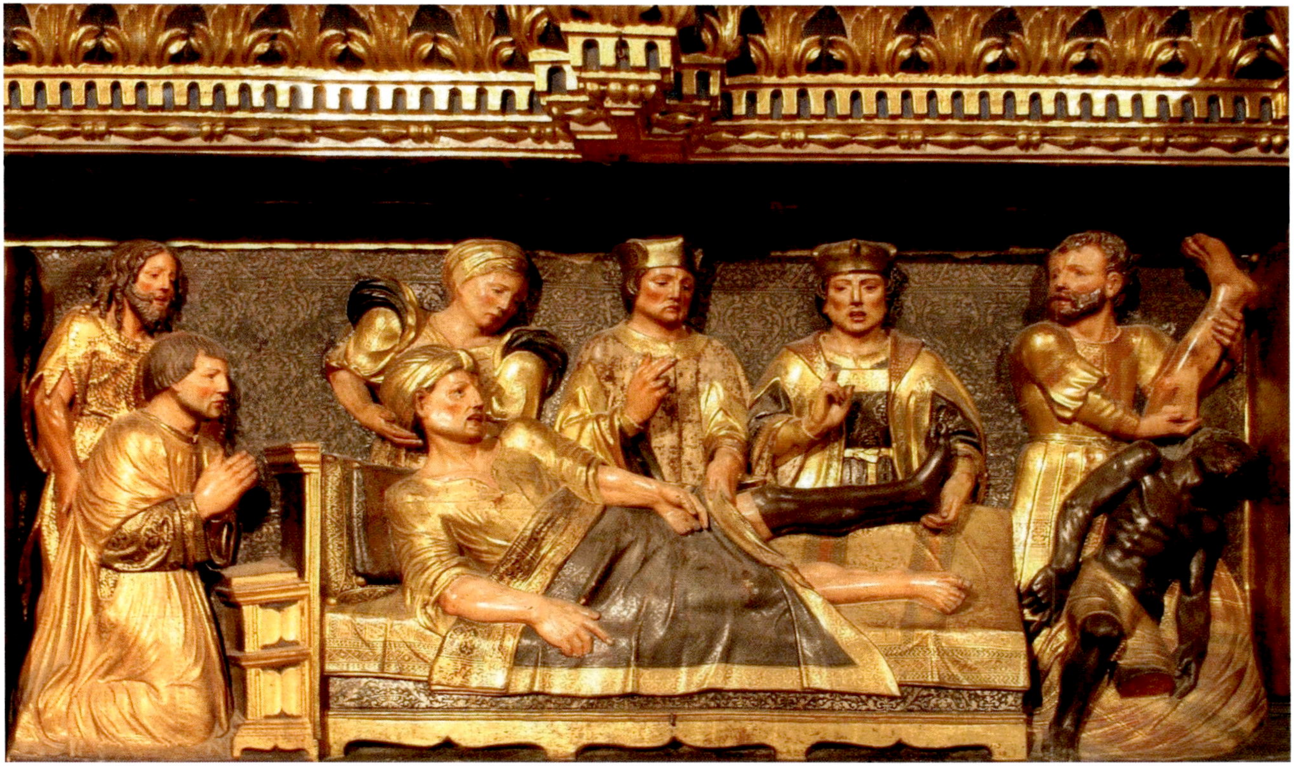

34. **Felipe Vigarny** (Langres, ca. 1470-1542, Toledo), *panel, polychrome woodcarving*, 1533.
Santa Iglesia Catedral de San Antolín, Palencia (Spain).

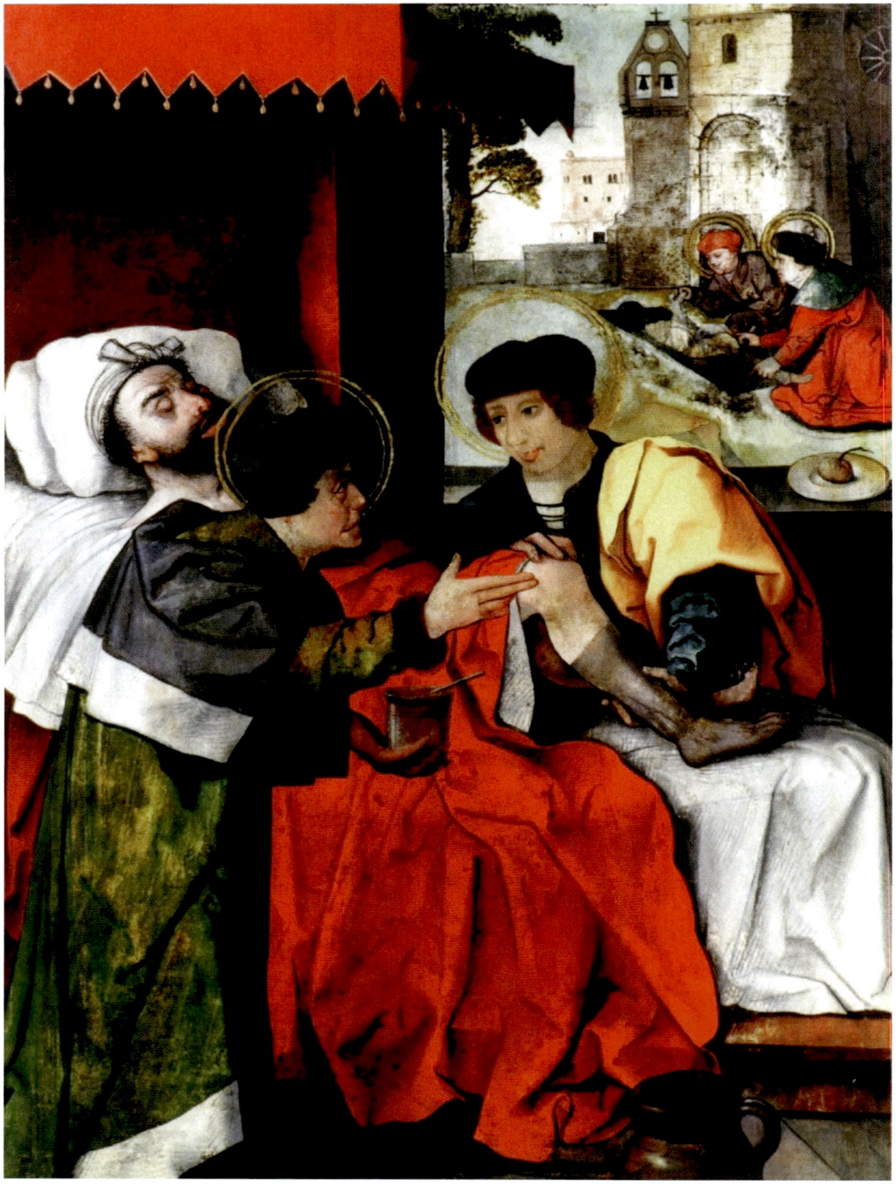

35. **Leon Picardo** (St.Omer, ?-1547, Burgos), *panel*, 1533. Museo Diocesano Catedralicio, Burgos (Spain).

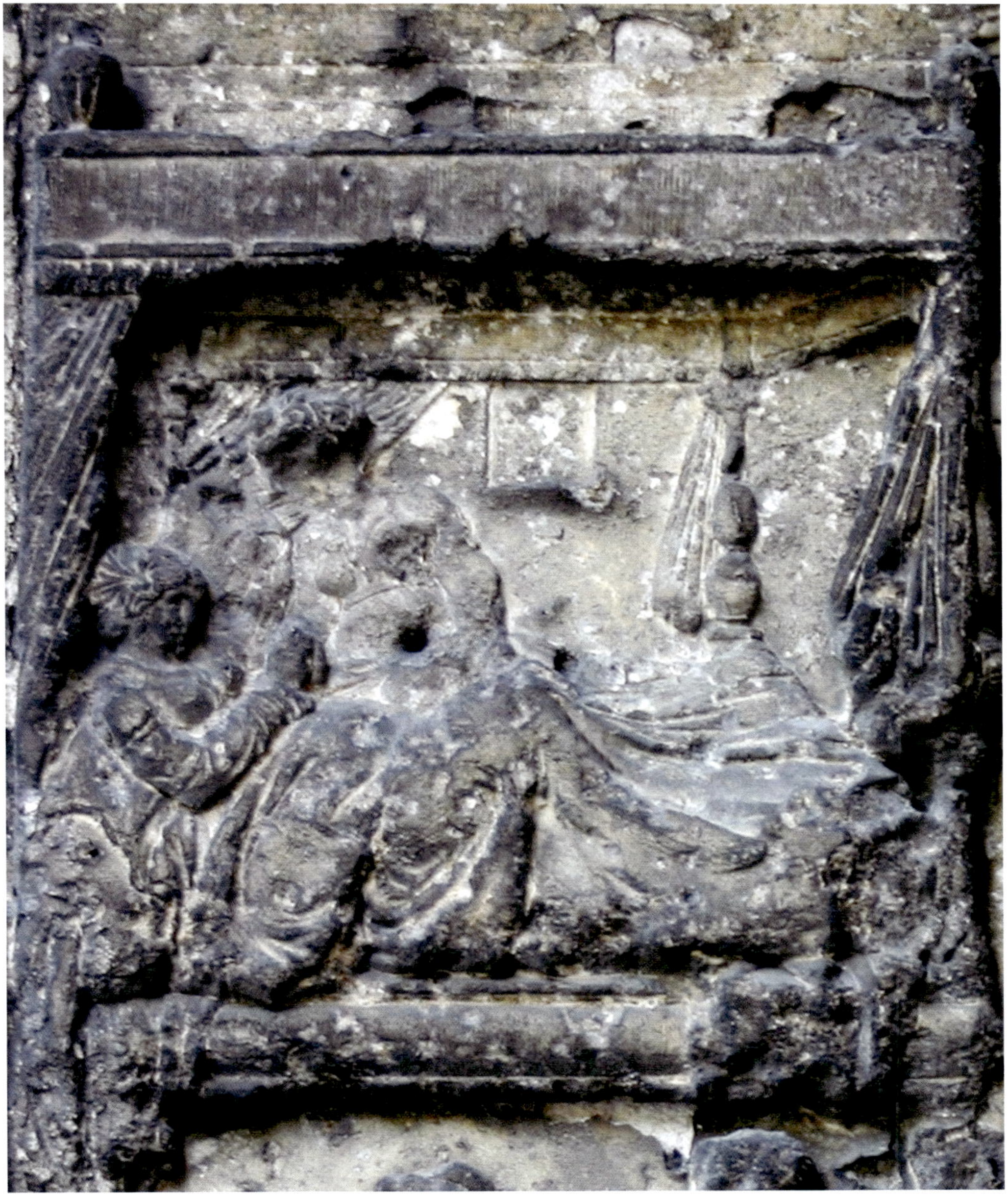

36. **Nicolas de Saint-Michel,** *sculpture in sandstone,* 1537. Église de Côme et Damien, Luzarches (France).

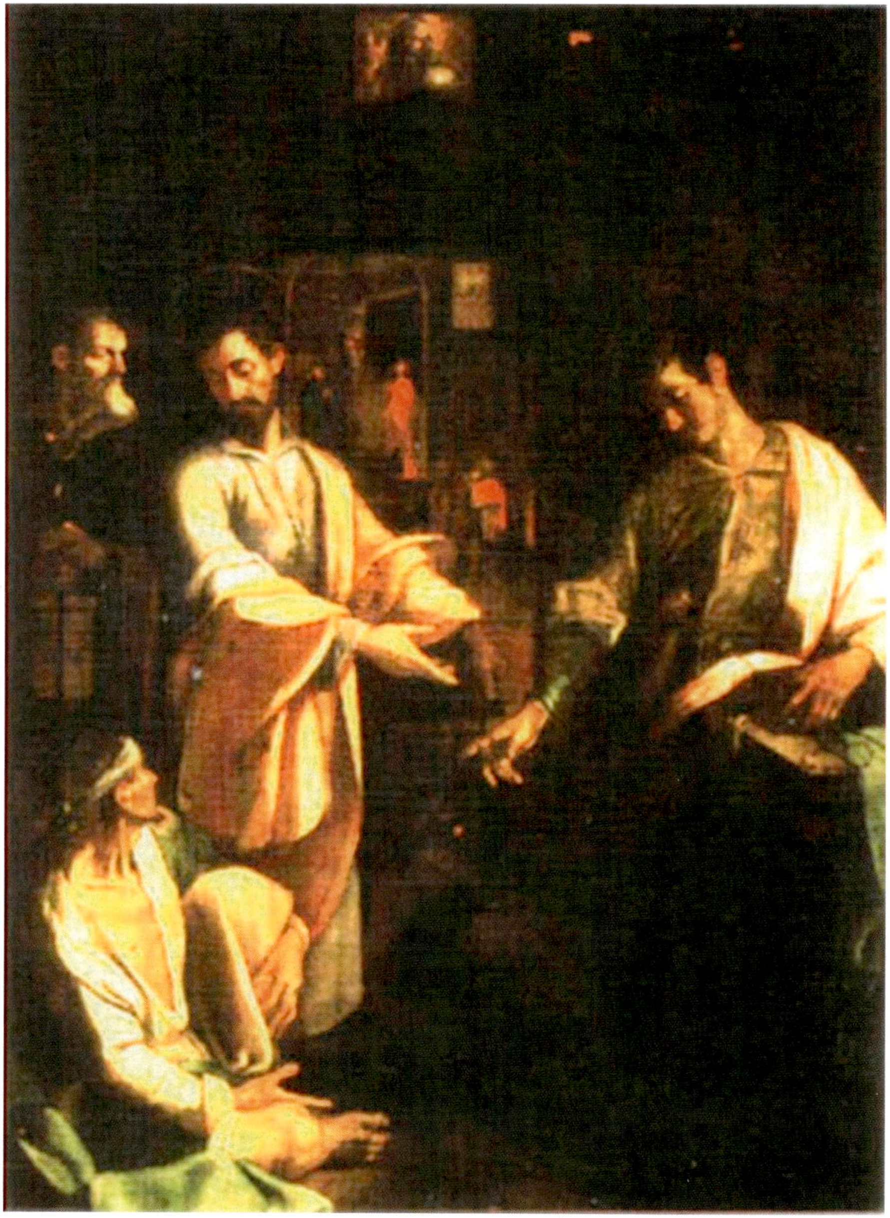

37. **Florentin Filippo Paladini** (1544-1616), *painting*. Church of St. Francis, Valletta (Malta).

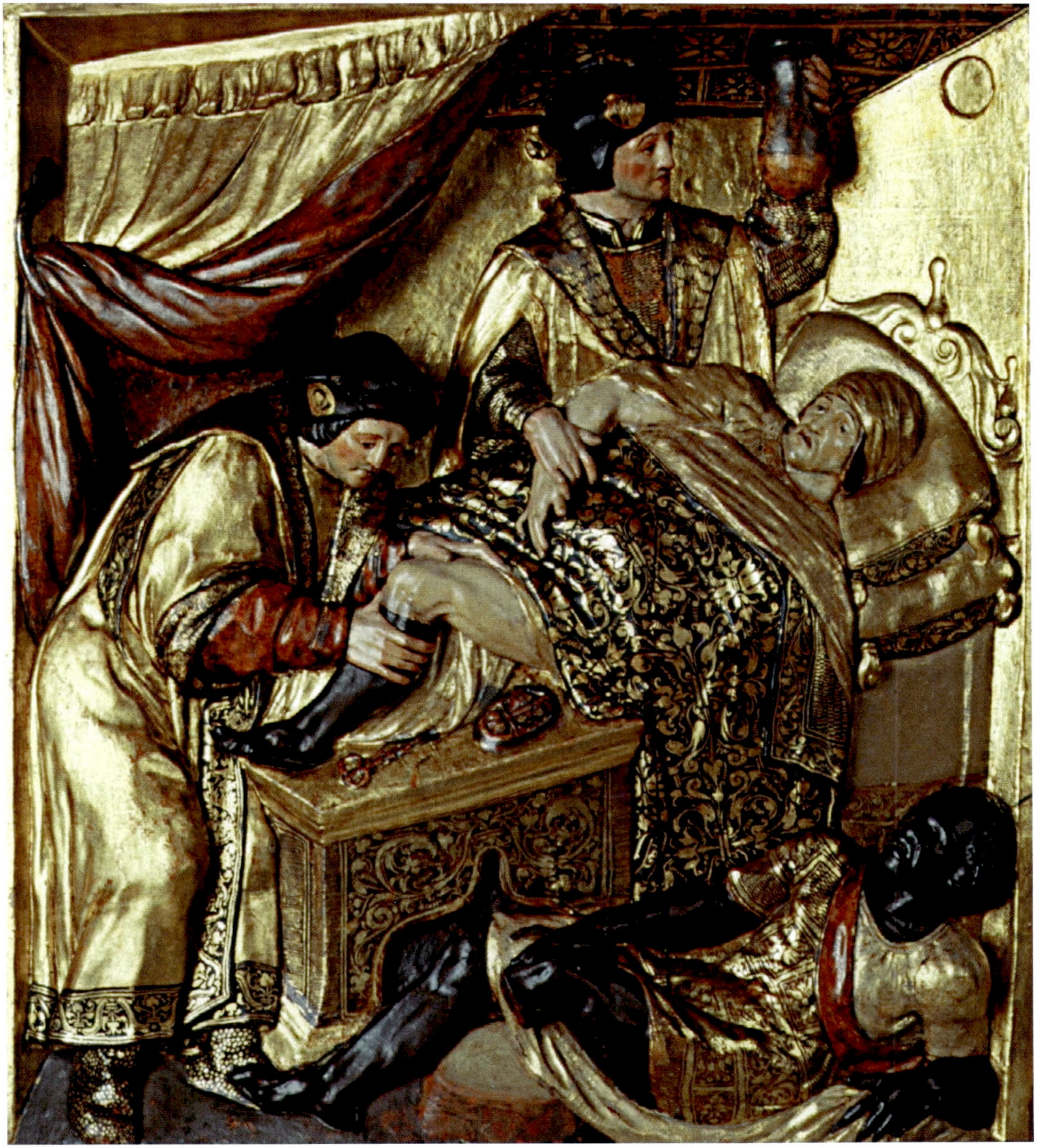

38. **Isidro Villoldo** (Toledo(?), ca. 1500-1556, Seville), *panel, polychrome woodcarving*, altarpiece for the S. Juana del Convento de S. Francisco, 1539 or 1547. Museo Nacional de Escultura, Valladolid (Spain).

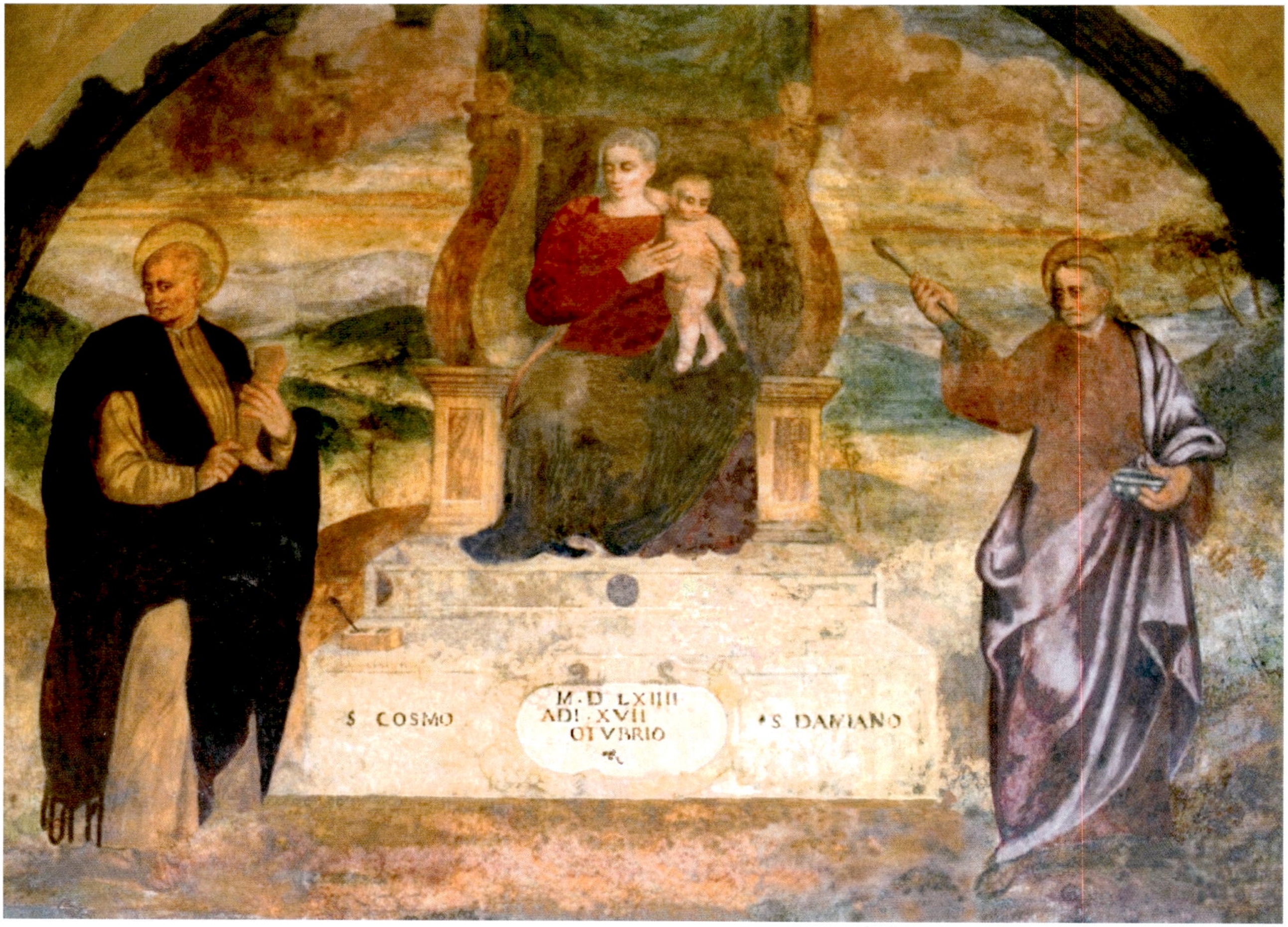

39. Antonio da Tisoi (ca.1485-1564), *fresco*, 1564. S. Rocco, Belluno (Italy).

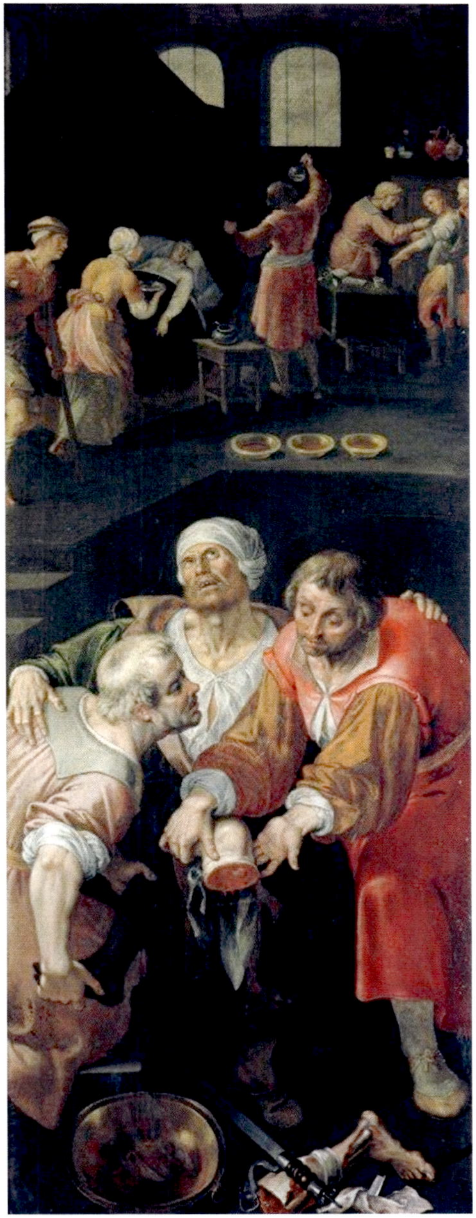

40. **Ambrosius Francken I** (Herentals, 1544-1618, Antwerpen), *panel (wing of an altarpiece),* 1590. Koninklijk Museum voor Schone Kunsten, Antwerpen (Belgium).

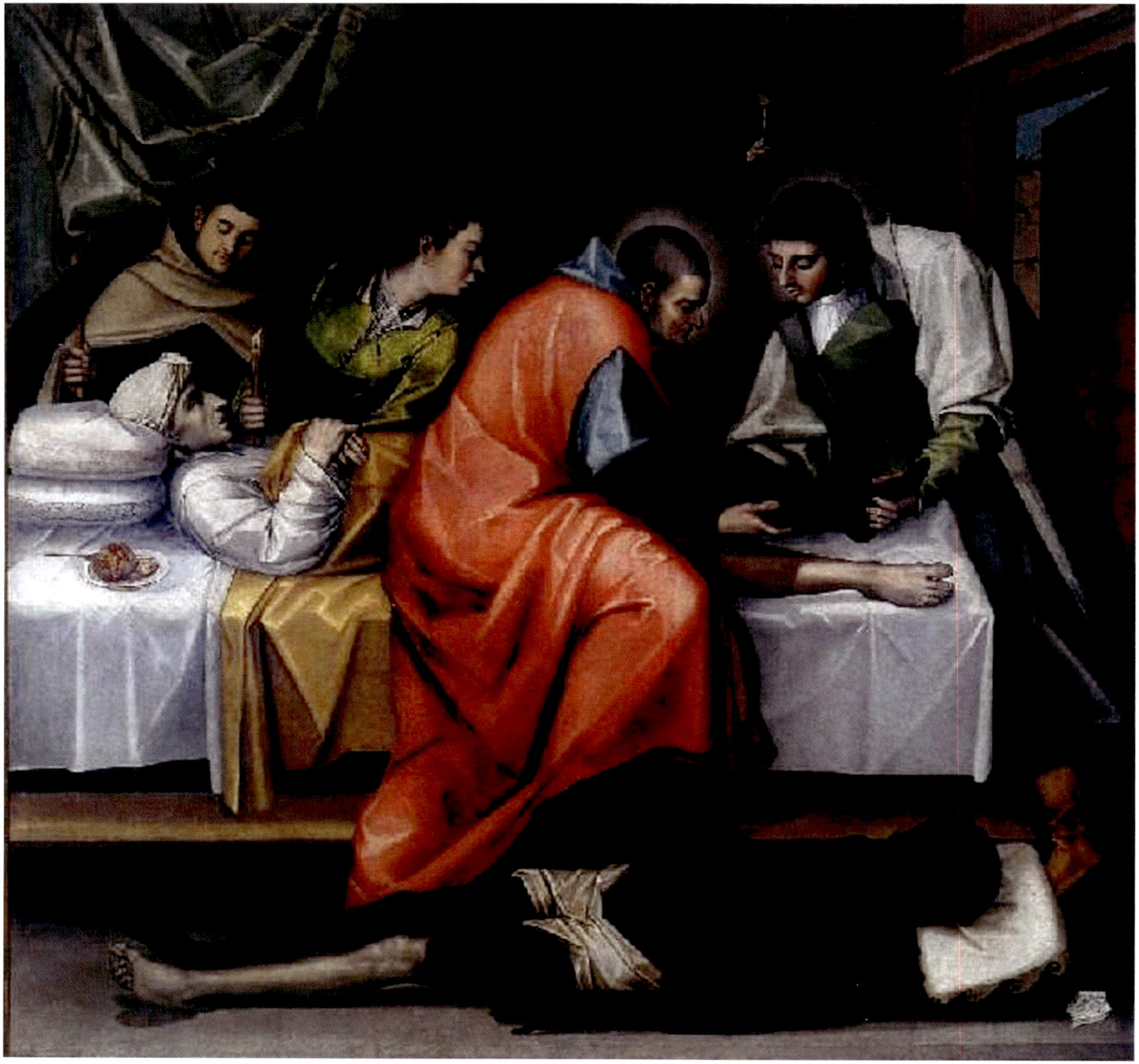

41. Pedro de Raxis (el Viego) (Alcalá de Henares, 1555-1626, Granada), *panel,* 1592. Museo de Bellas Artes, Granada (Spain).

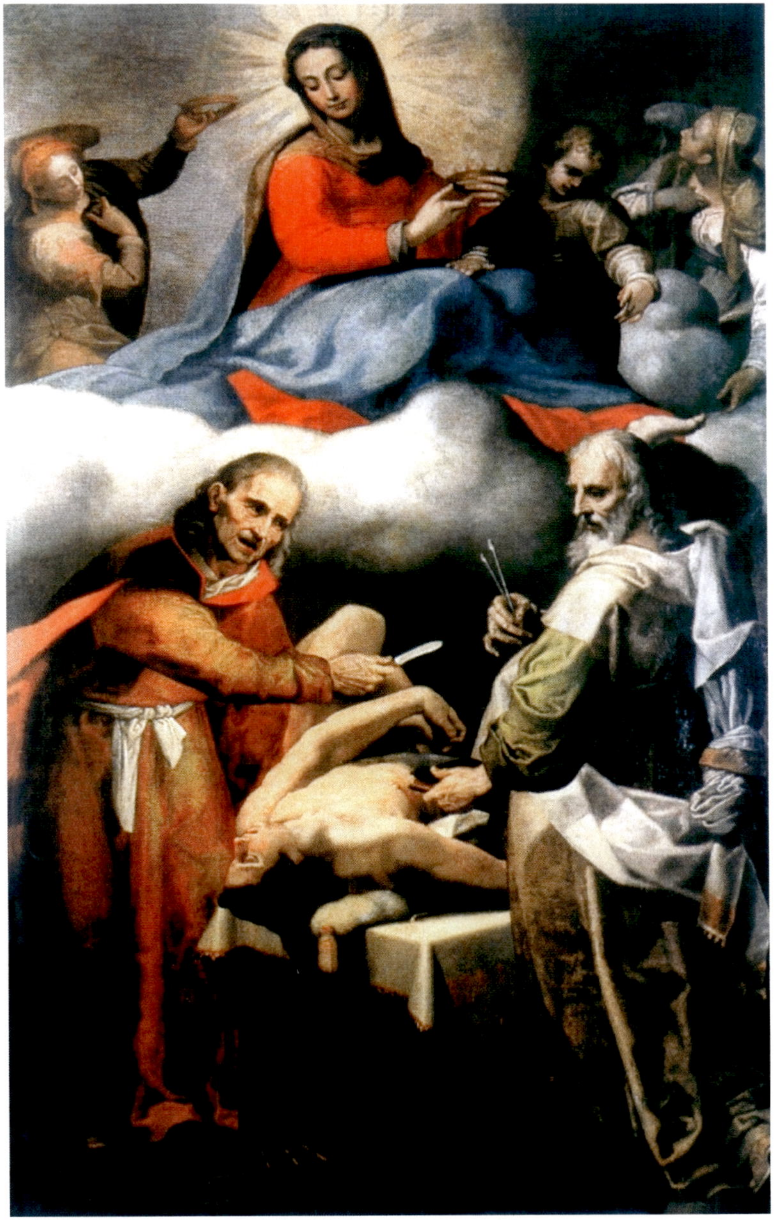

42. **Giovanni Battista Tinti** (Parma, 1558-1604, Parma), *painting,* 1594. Galleria Nazionale di Parma, 'su concessione del Ministero per I Beni Culturali', Parma (Italy).

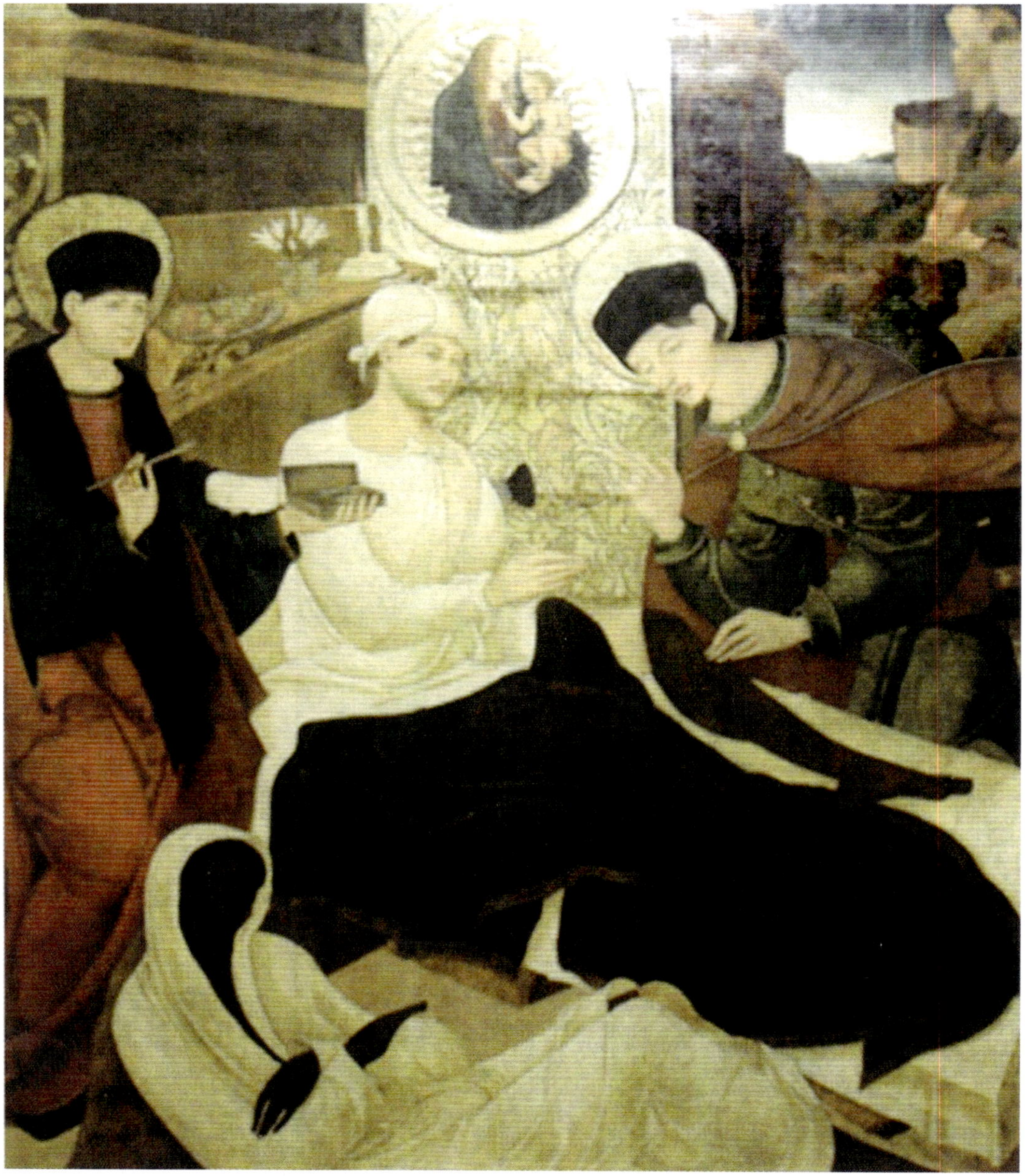

43. **unknown,** *painting?,* 16th century (?). Whereabouts unknown (Spain?).

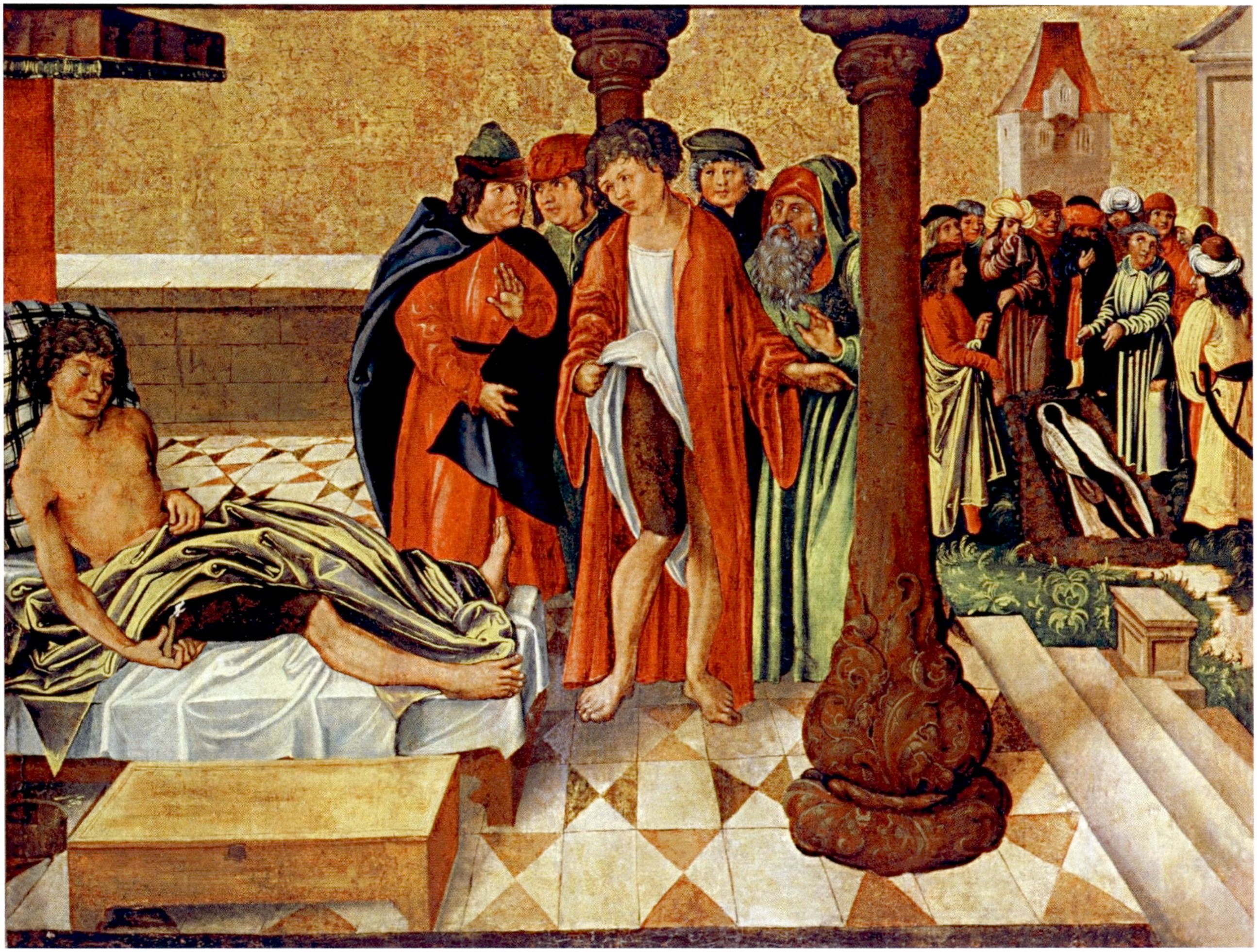

44. **"Master of the Legend Scenes",** *panel, transferred to canvas,*
early 16th century. Österreichische Galerie Belvedere, Vienna (Austria).

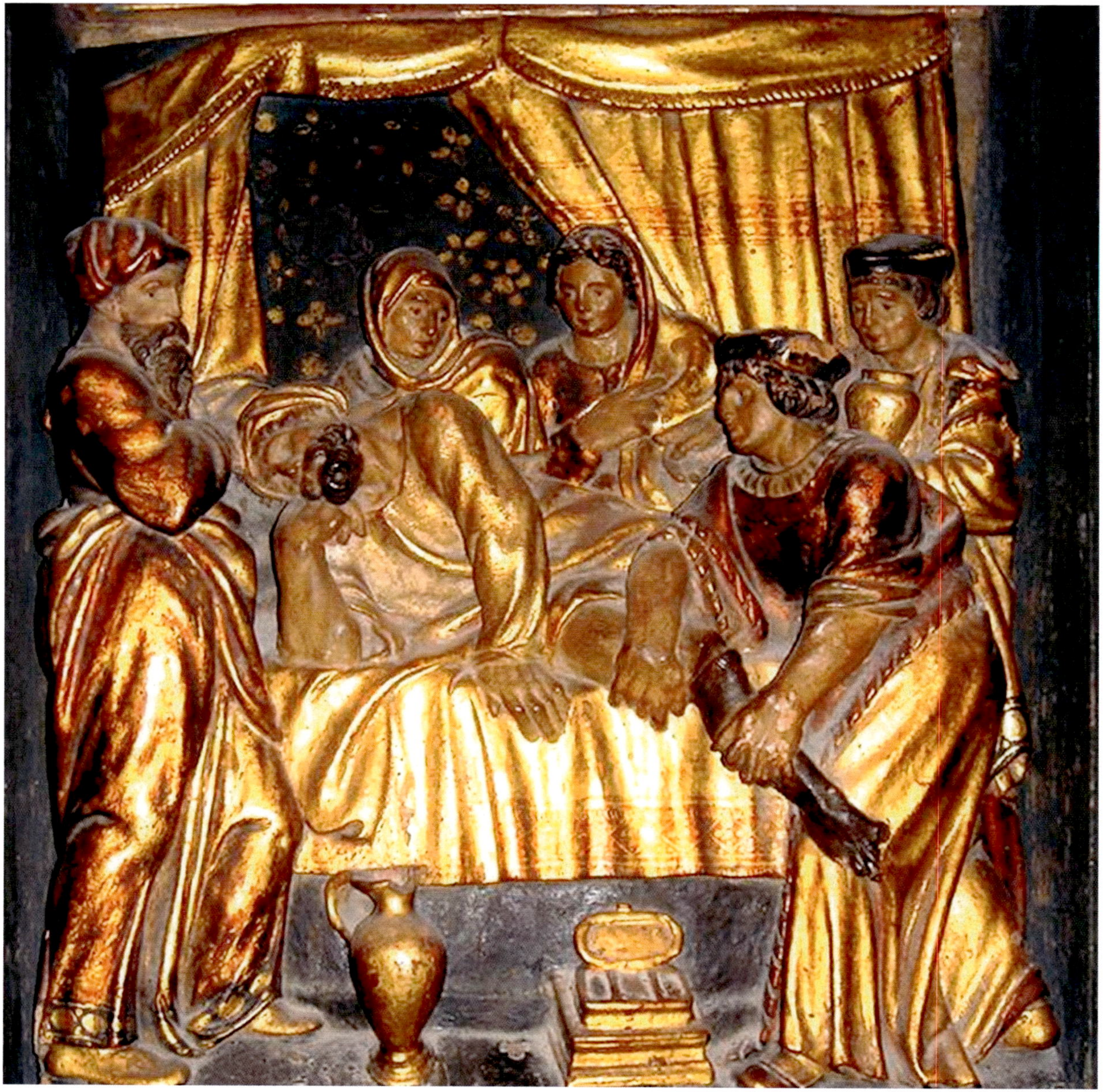

45. **Anonymous,** *panel of altarpiece, polychrome woodcarving,* 16th century. S. Pedro, Teruel (Spain).

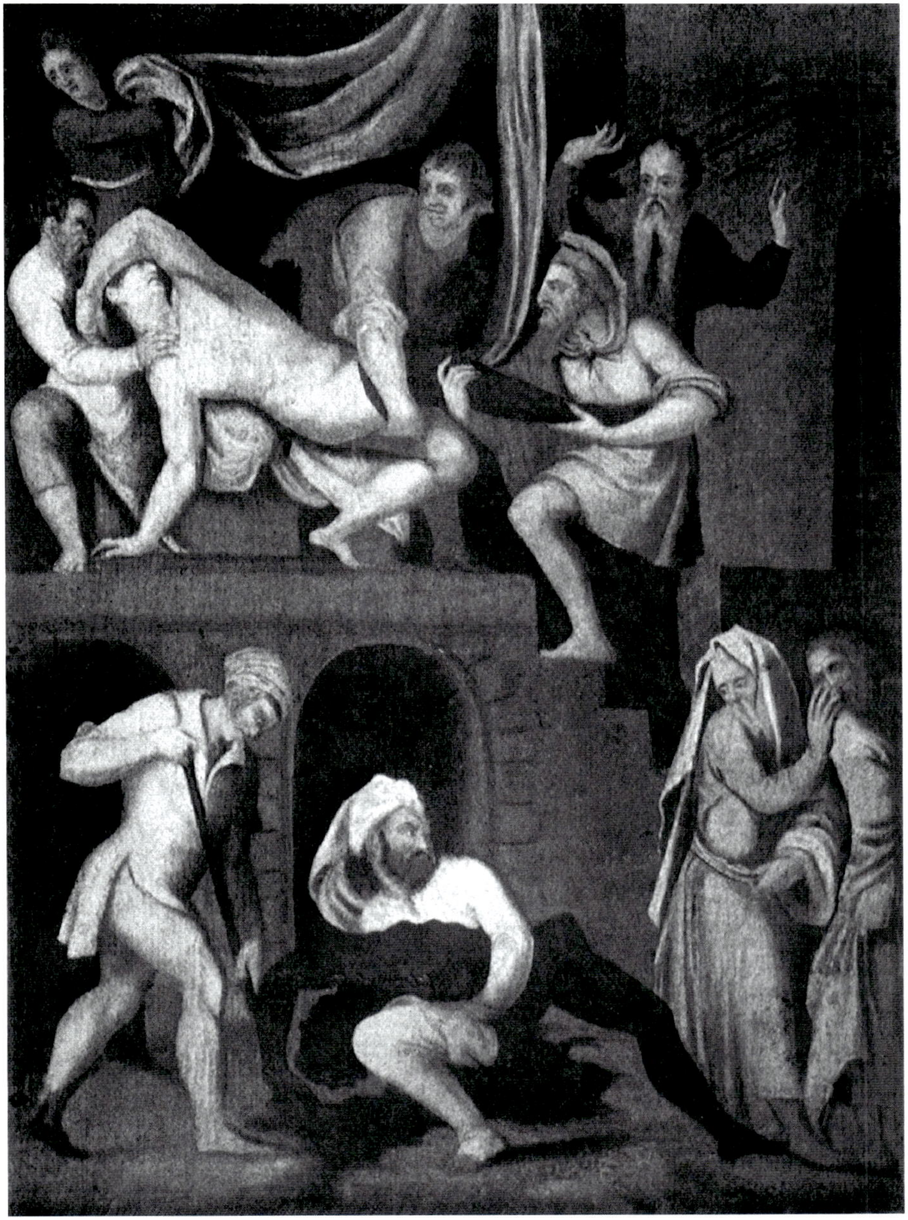

46. **Anonymous,** *painting*, 16th century. Whereabouts unknown (France? Formerly in the collection of M. Louis Forest).

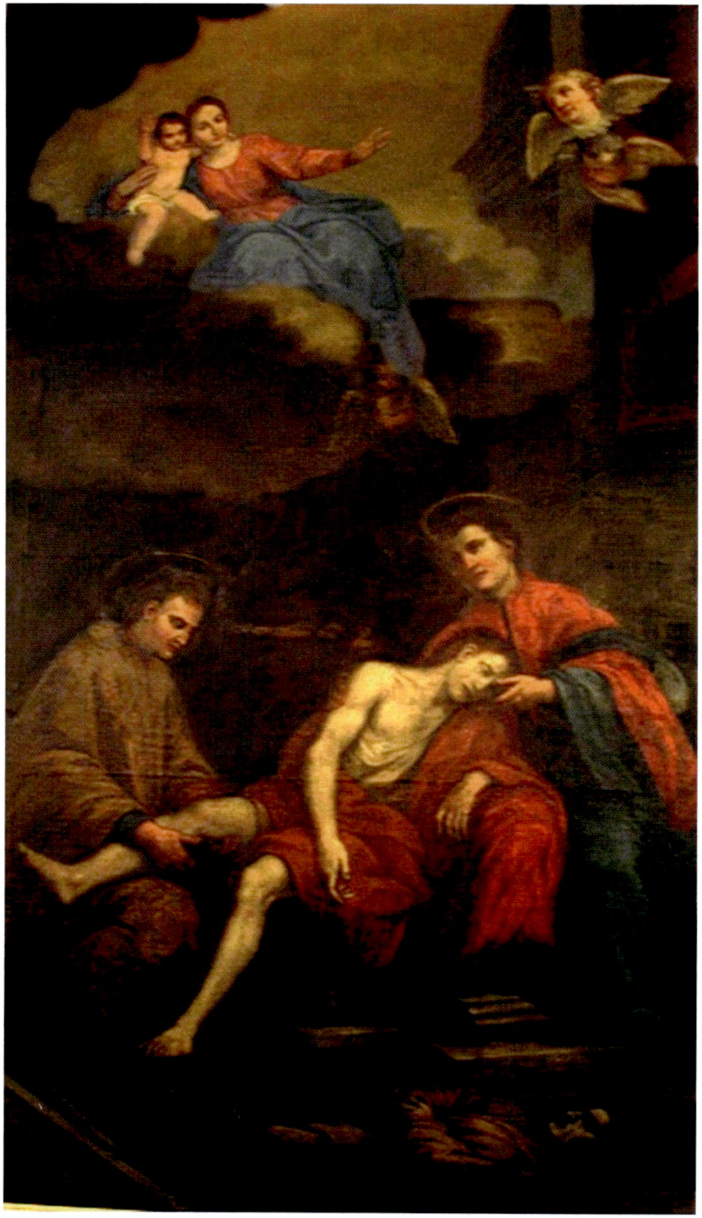

47. Bartolomeo Ramenghi (Bagnacavallo, 1484-1542, Bologna), *canvas*, 16th century. Chiesa di SS. Cosma e Damiano, Pegola (Italy)

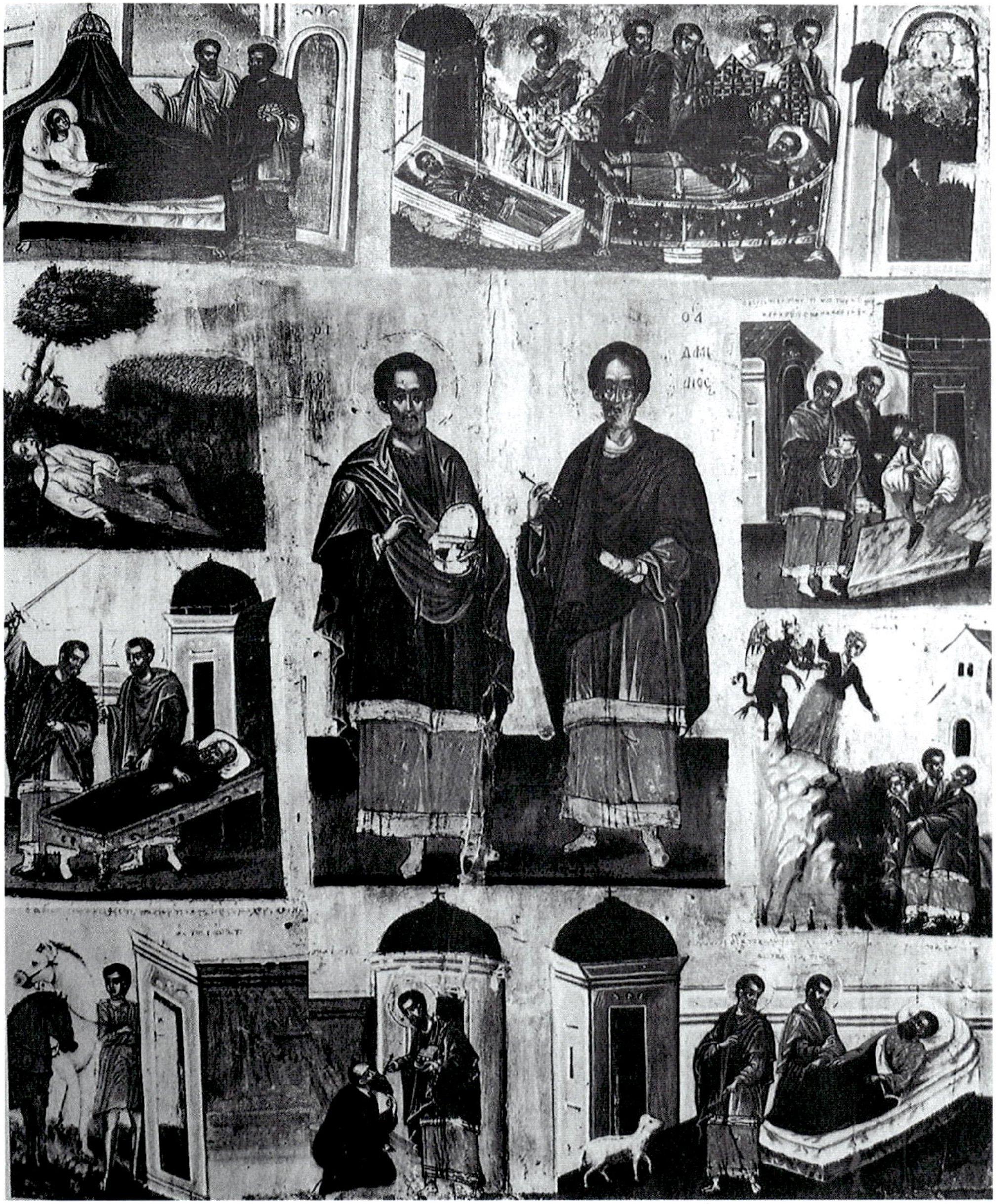

48. **Emanuele Tzanfornaris** (1570-1631), *icon,* 1600. Museo delle Icone, Chiesa di S. Giorgio dei Greci, Venice (Italy)

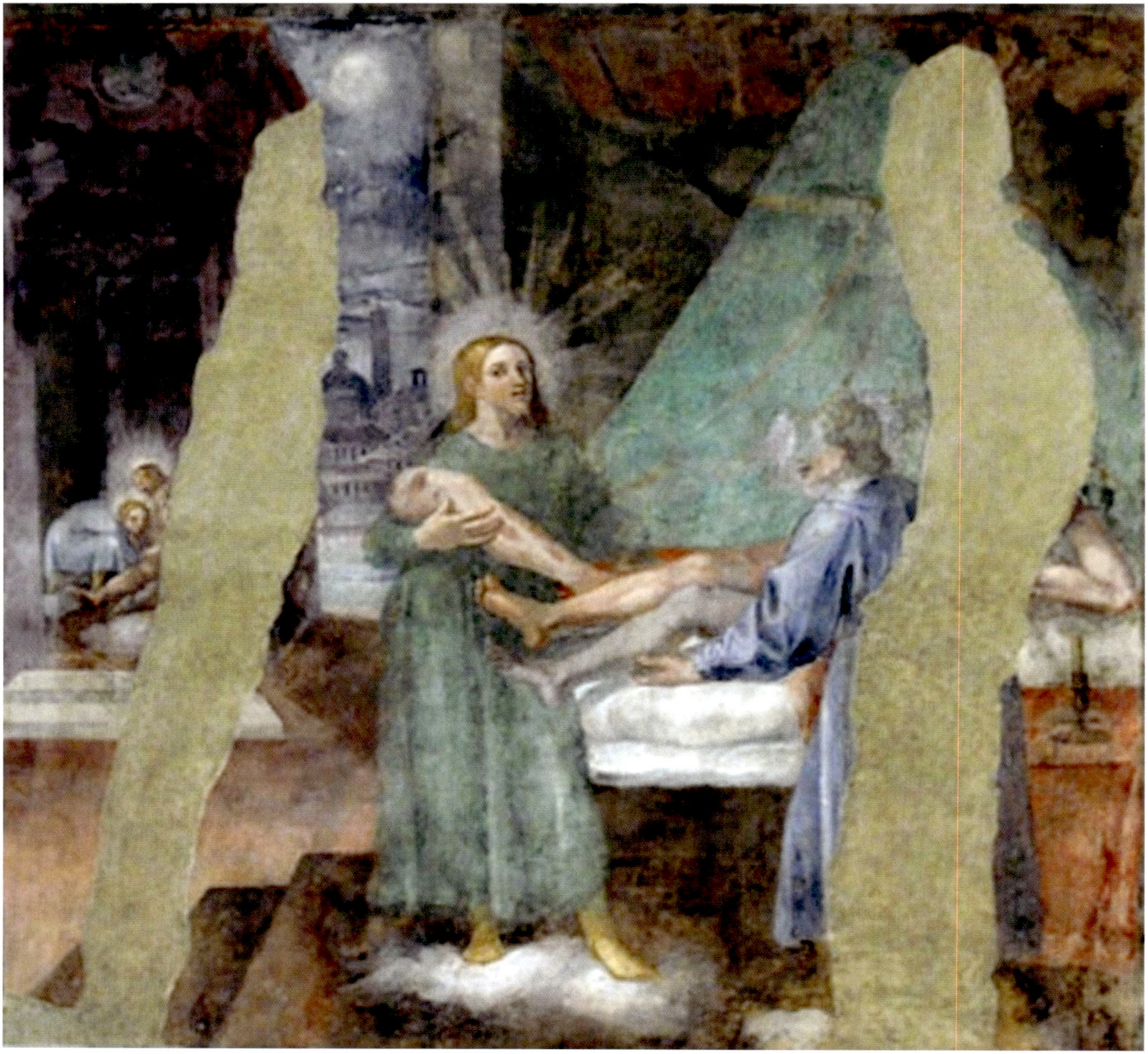

49. Agostino Beltrano and Agostino Pussé, *fresco*, 1639. Chiesa dei Santi Cosma e Damiano, Isernia (Italy).

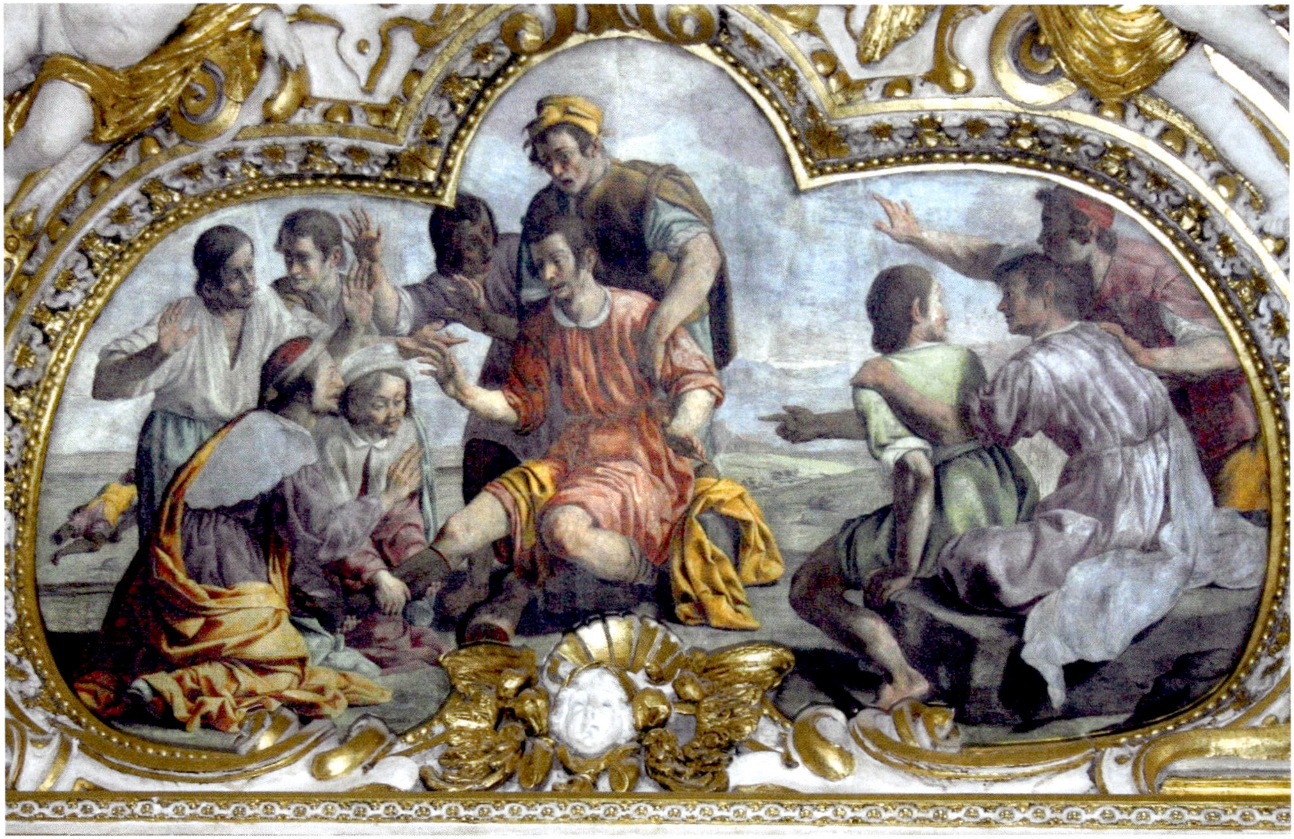

50. **Paolo Domenico Finoglia** (1590-1645), *ceiling painting*, ca.1630. Chiesa di Santi Cosma e Damiano, Conversano (Italy).

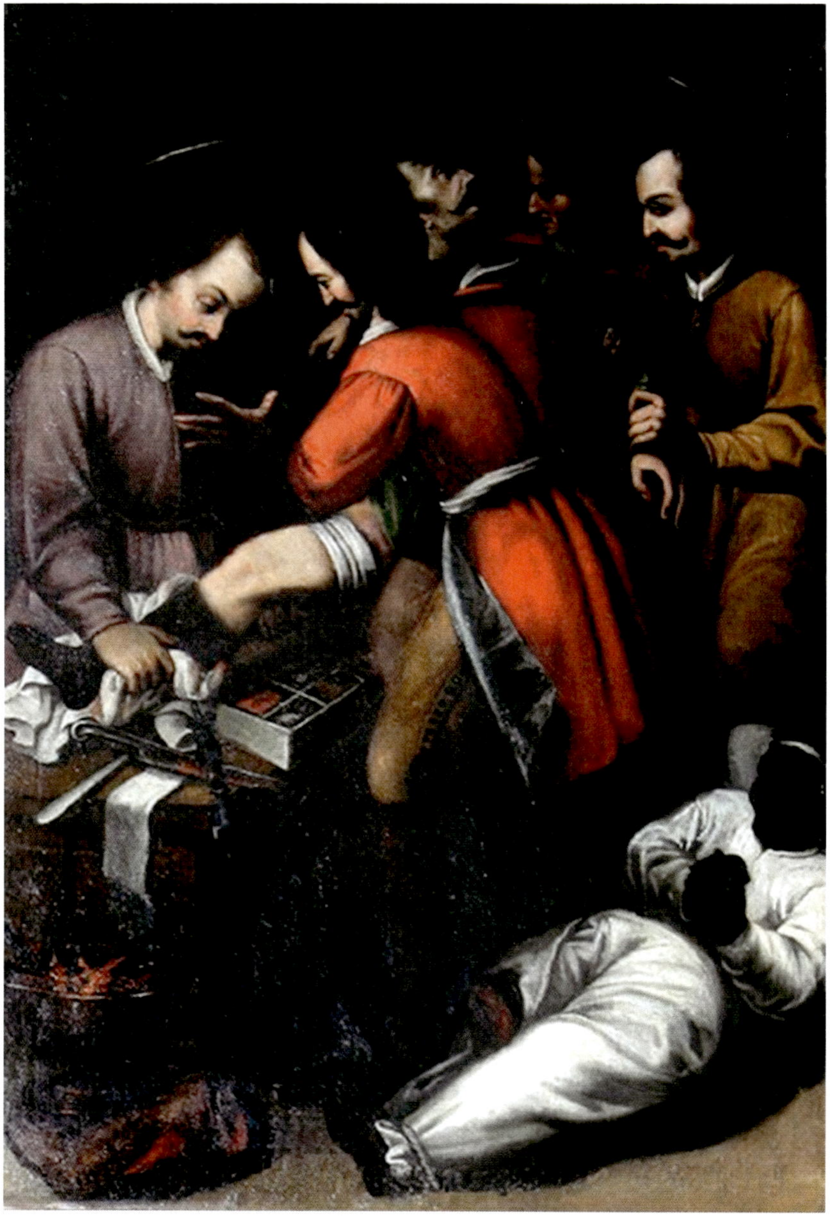

51. **Anonymous,** *painting*, 1657. Capilla de la Universidad, Sevilla (Spain).

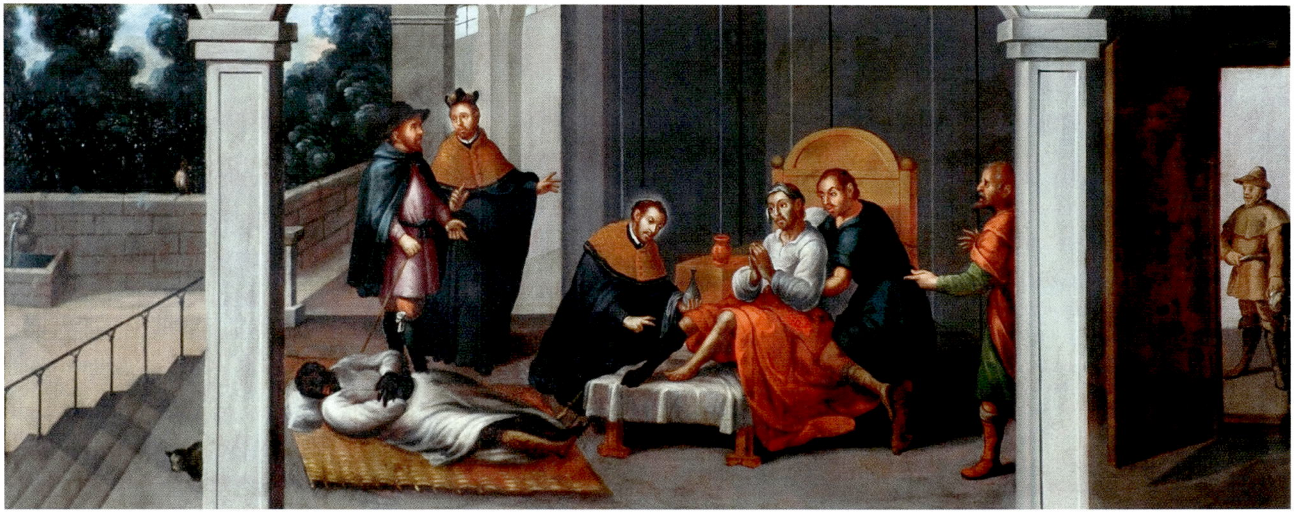

52. **Sebastián López Dávalos** (Puebla, ca. 1615-ca. 1694, Mexico city), *panel (predella scene)*, 1666. Catedral Mexico city, (Mexico).

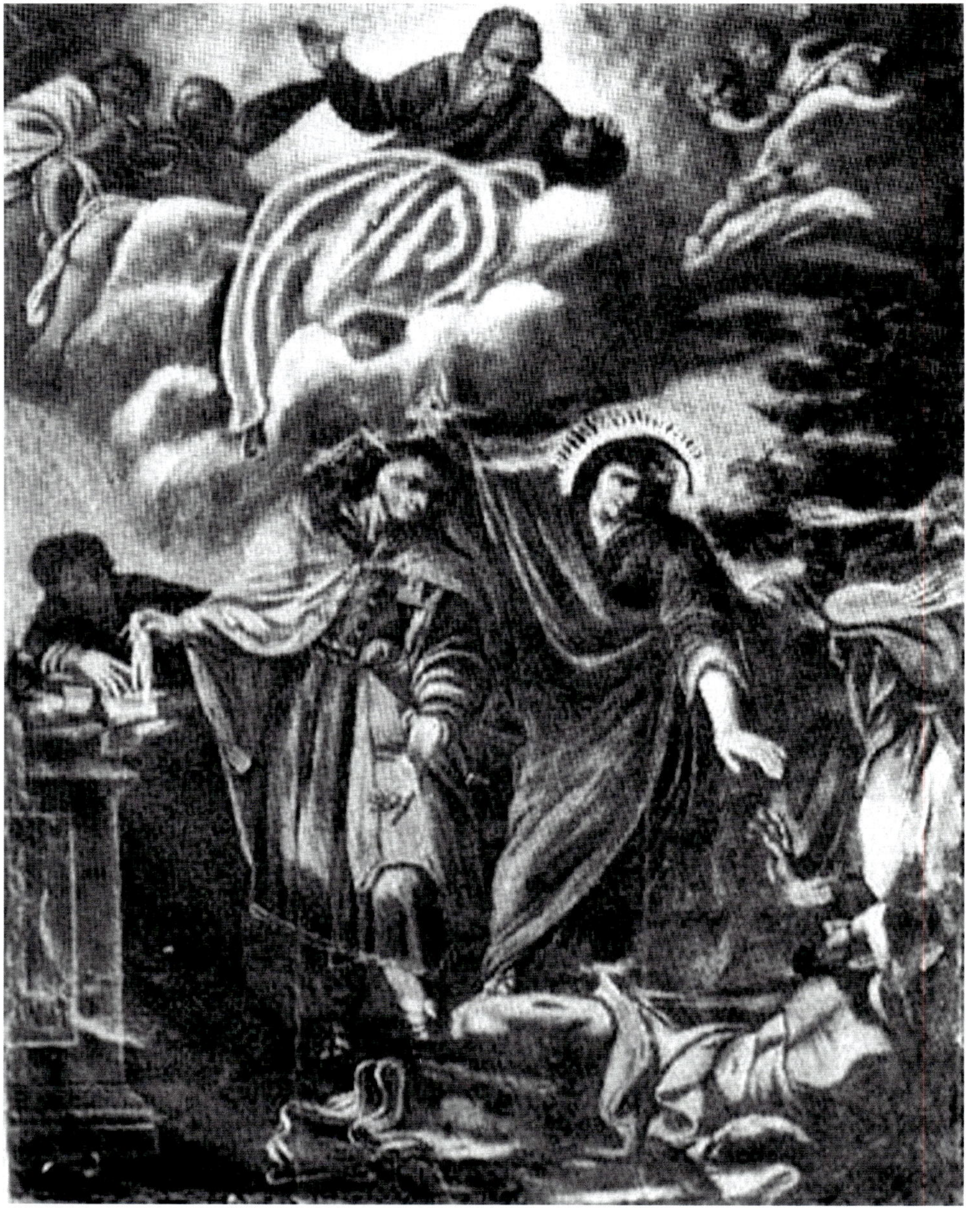

53. **Anonymous,** *painting,* 1688. Chiesa di Gesù e Maria, Pantheon, Paterno (Italy).

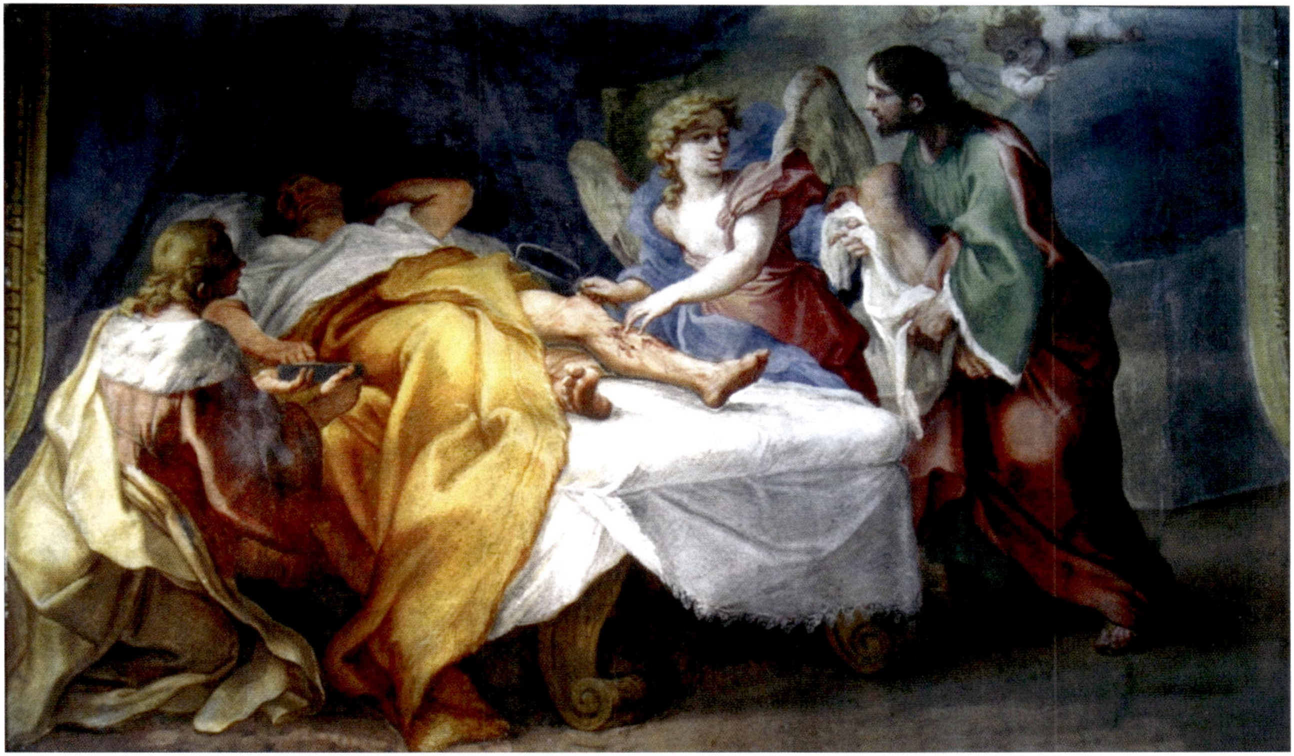

54. **Stefano Maria Legnani ("Legnanino")** (Milano, 1661-1713, Milano), *wall painting*, 1691. Chiesa Santi Cosma e Damiano, Uboldo (Italy).

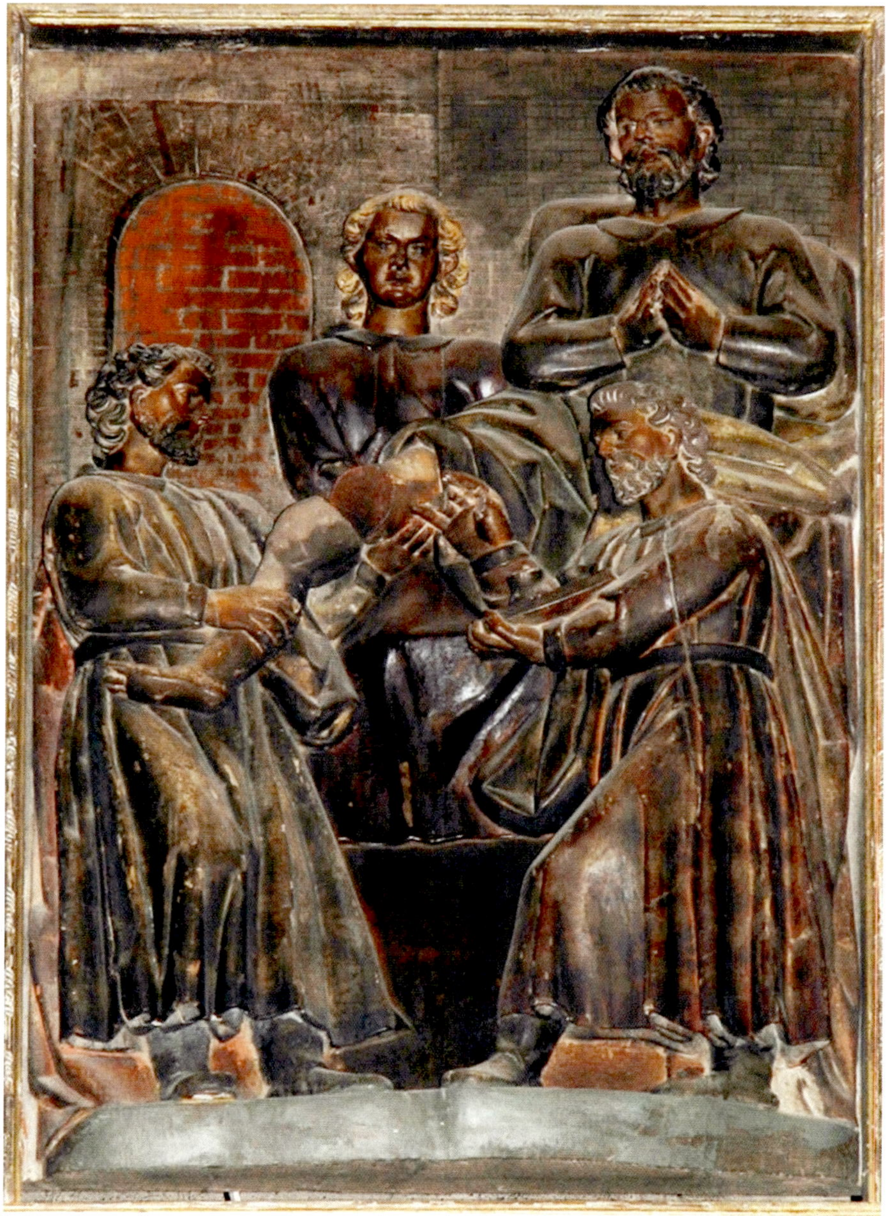

55. **José Rodríguez, Mateo de Olmos and Pedro de Cicarte,** *panel of altarpiece,* 17th century (?). Iglesia de Cosme y Dámian, Hontoria del Pinar (Spain).

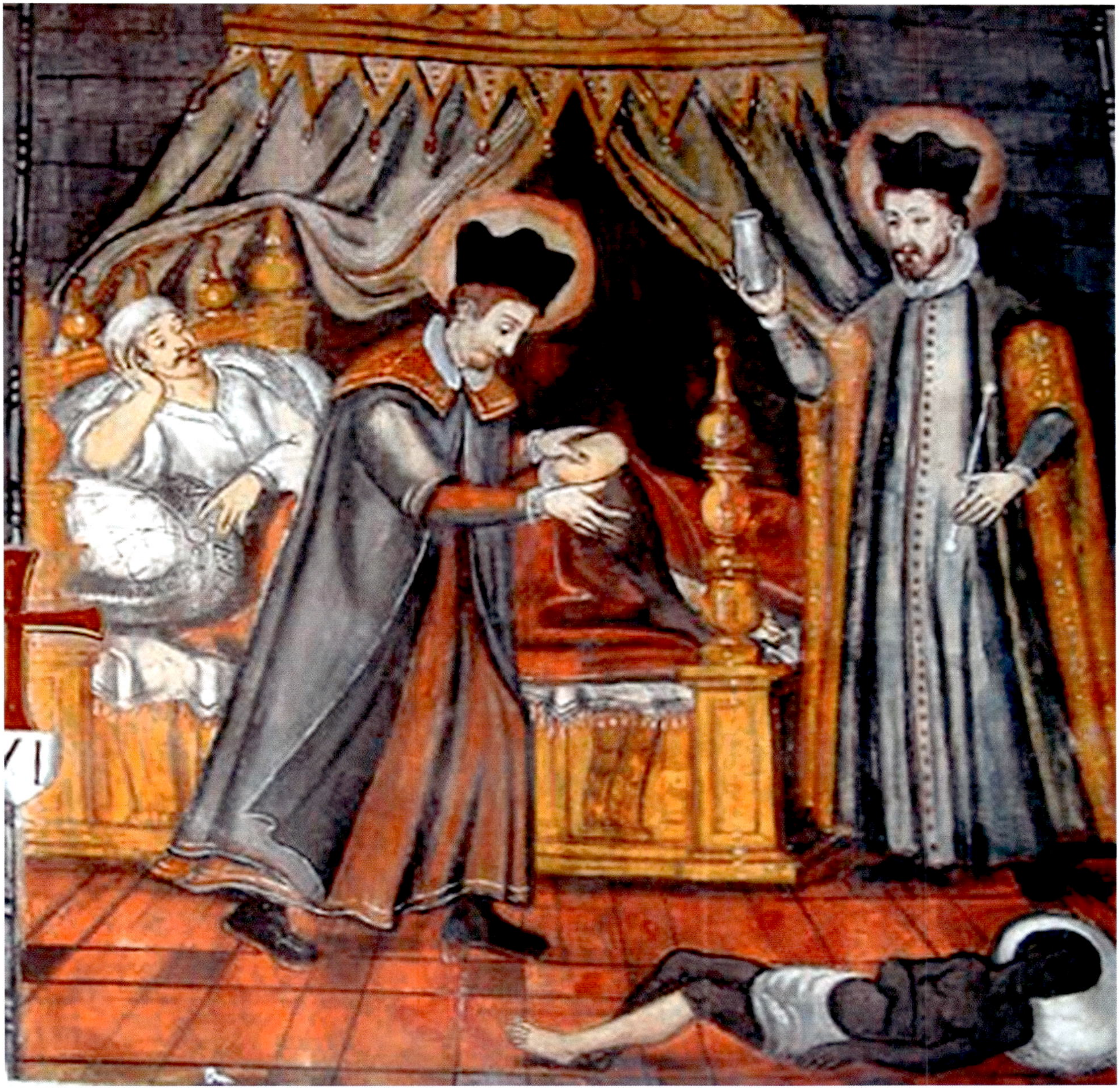

56. **Anonymous,** *panel*, 17th century. Santuario de Santa Eulalia de Mérida, Totana (Spain).

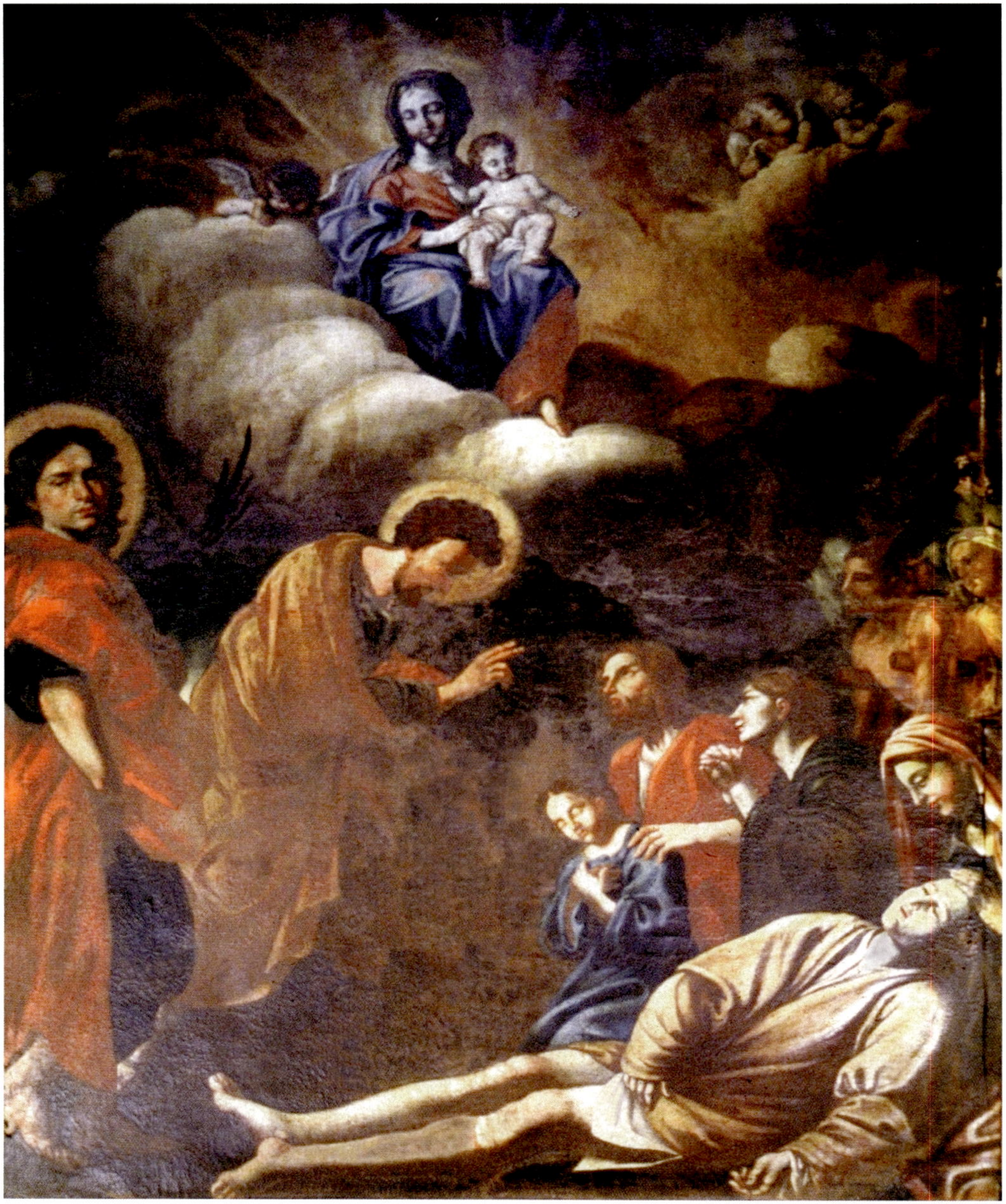

57. **Anonymous,** *canvas,* 17th century. Chiesa Parrocchiale di Santi Cosma e Damiano, Grazzano Visconti (Italy).

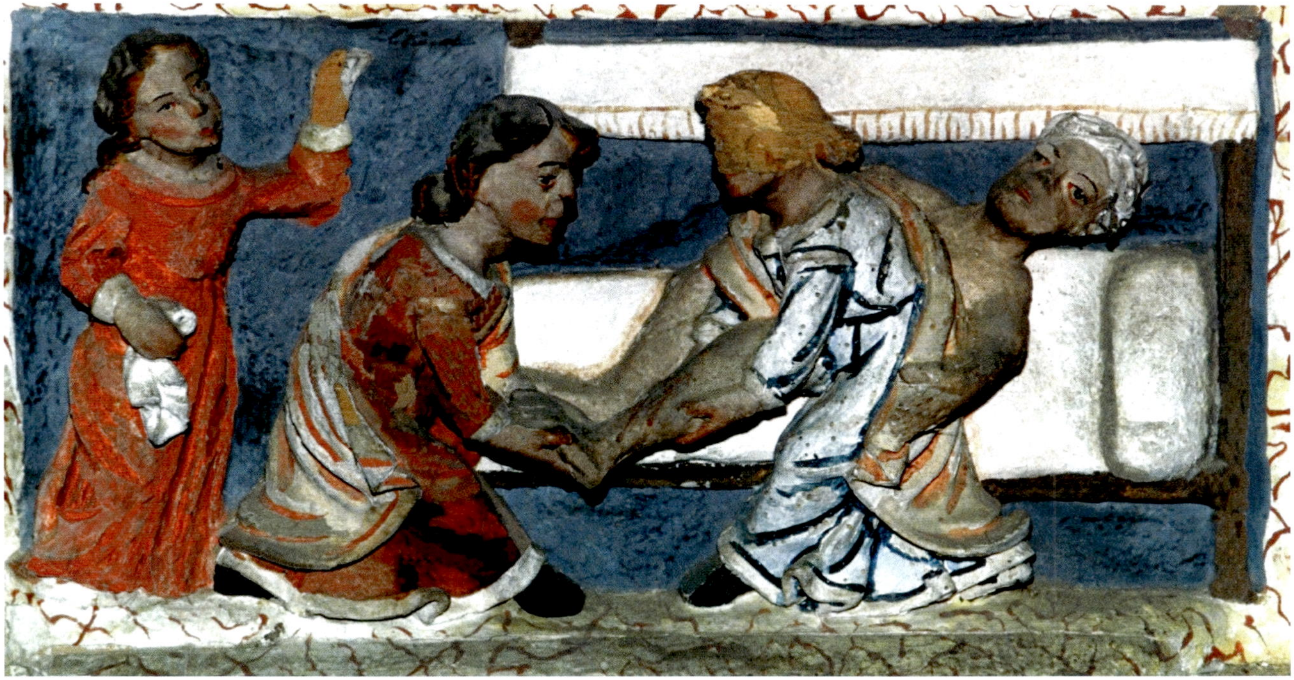

58. **Anonymous,** *panel of altarpiece, polychrome woodcarving,* 1723. Chapelle Saint Côme et Saint Damien, La Llau (France).

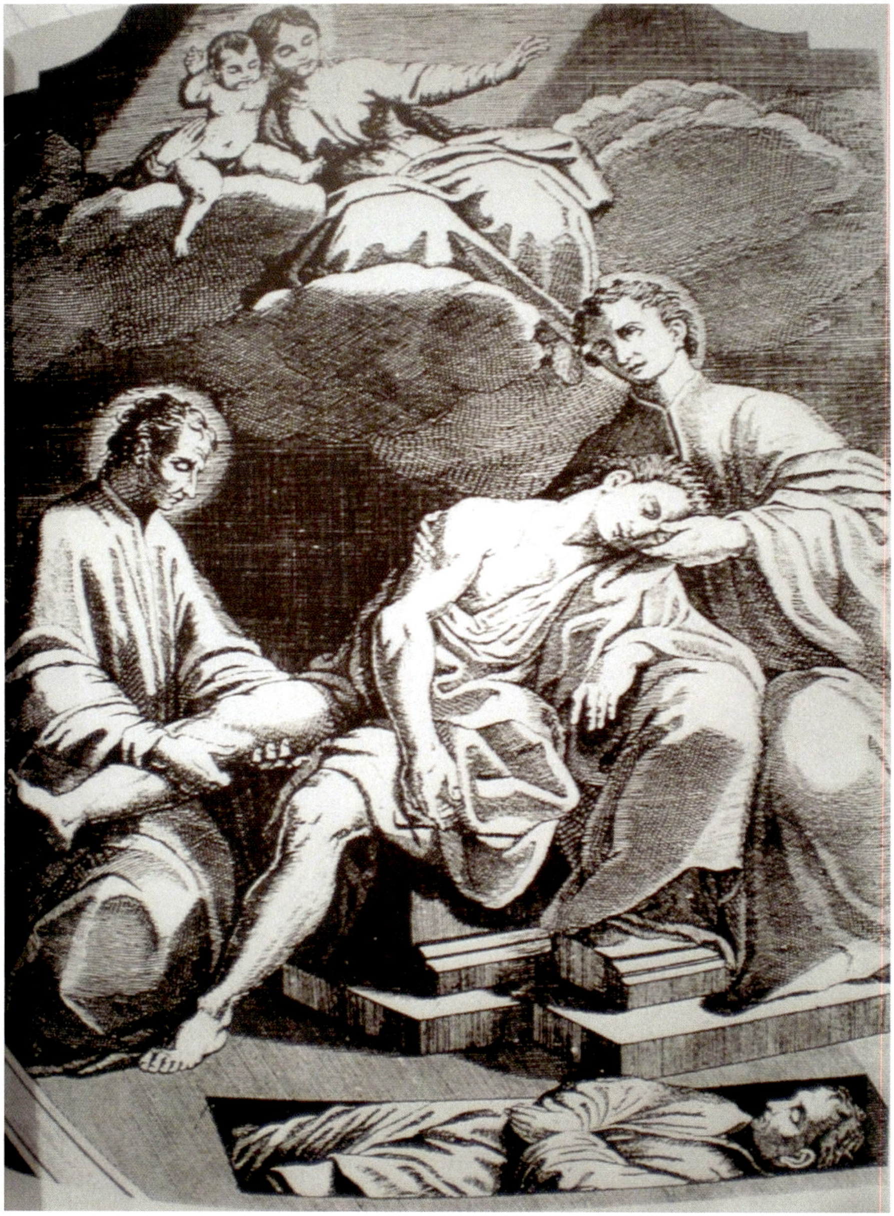

59. **Michele Benedetti,** *etching,* 1750. Archiginnasio, Bologna (Italy).

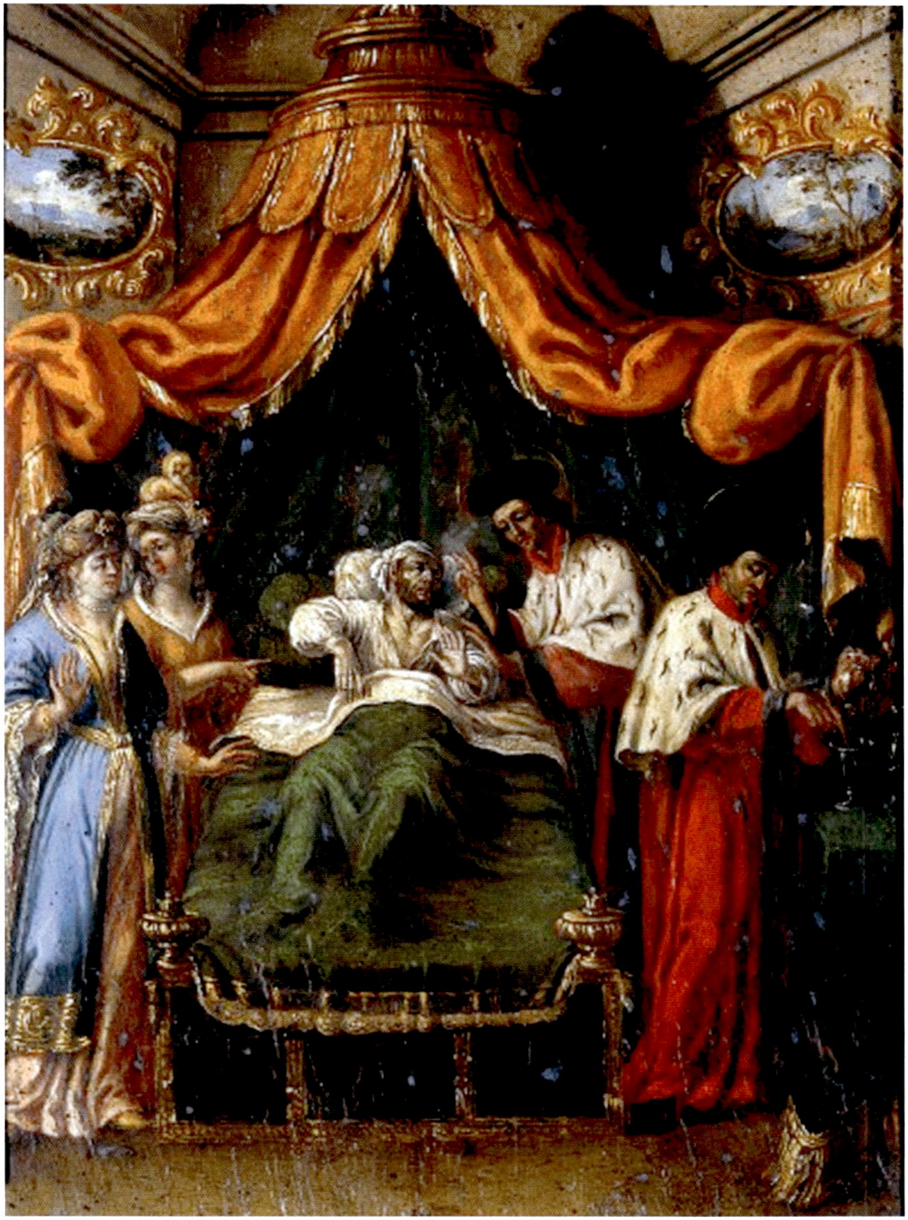

60. **Anonymous,** *canvas,* 18th century. Wellcome Library (nr. 44845i), London (UK).

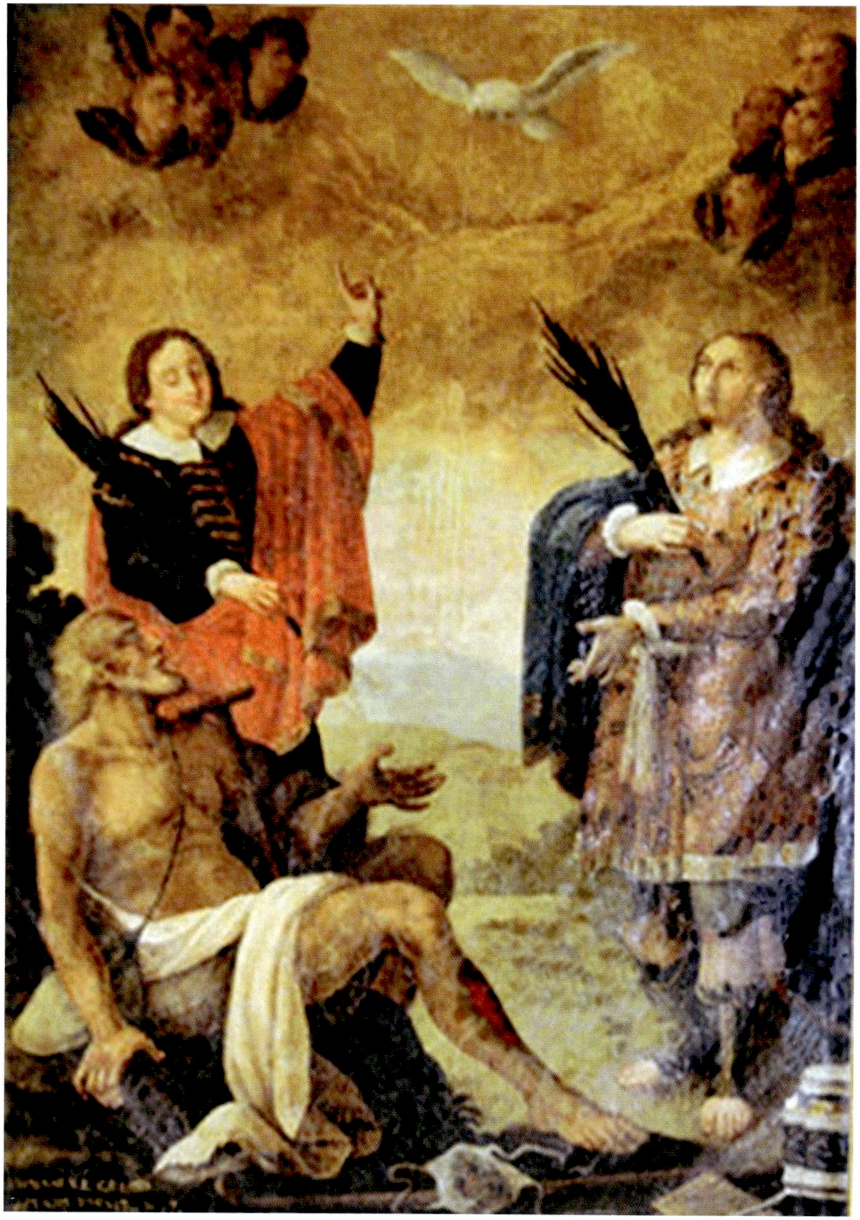

61. **Grossonaso,** *canvas*, 1827. Chiesa S. Antonio Abate Emanuele, Pedara (Italy).

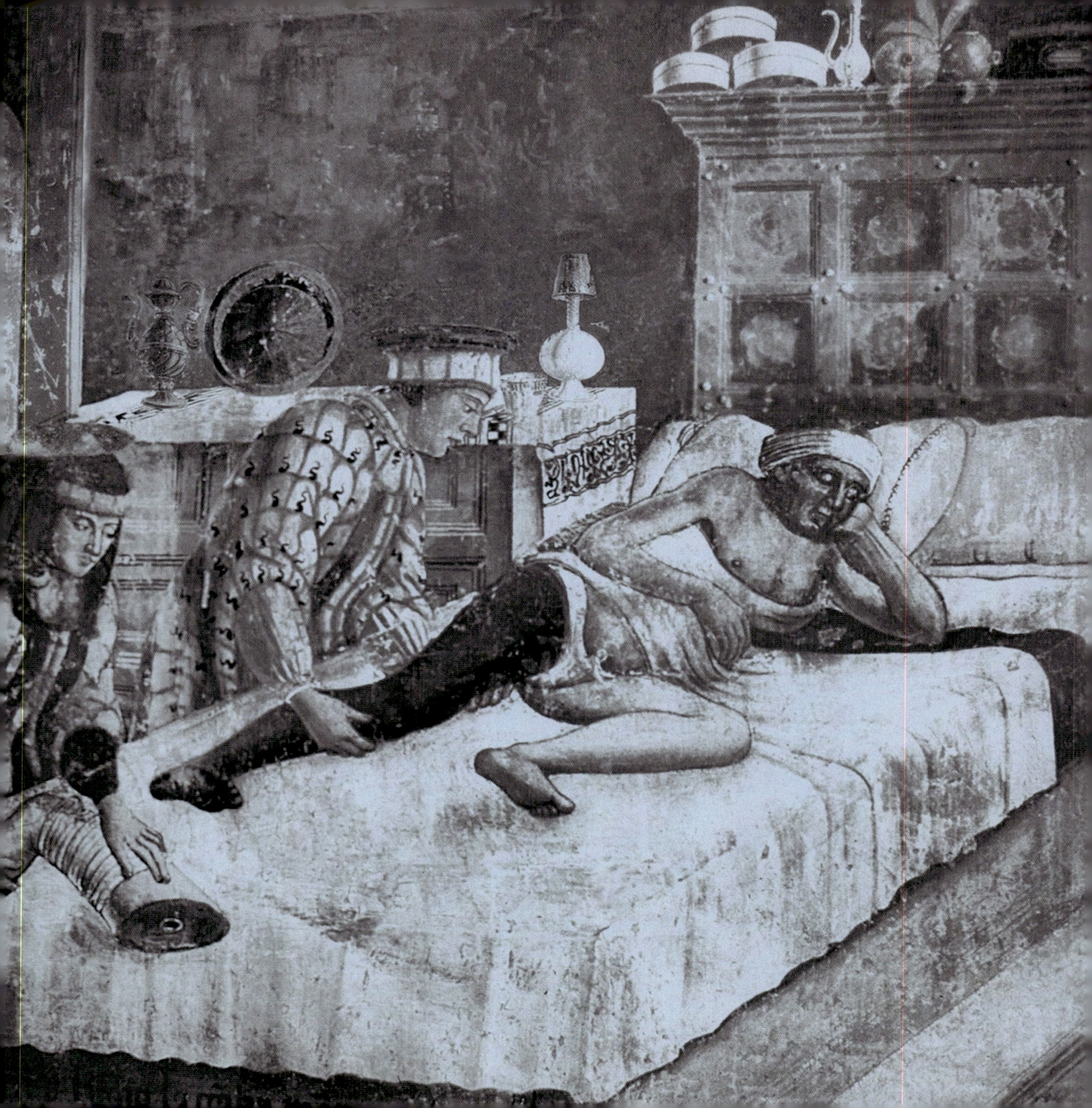

Cosmas and Damian as representatives of a diverse medical profession and its functions

Catrien G. Santing

The Martinikerk in Groningen, dedicated to St Martin, has a fifteenth-century vault painting of the twin medical doctors and saints Cosmas and Damian (Ill. IV page 25). The scene differs substantially from the focus on amputation in this book as there is no severed leg to be seen. Mother Mary is flanked by the brothers, with Saint Cosmas on her left clothed in the full dress of the learned *medicinae doctor*, wearing a doctor's hat and holding up a full urinal, while on her right his brother Damian stands in the short-robed attire of the artisan surgeon with a medicine box and what looks like a lancet or a spatula in his hands. Both are provided with a sword, which indicates their martyrdom and bears no relation to the amputation miracle under scrutiny in this book. Thus, in this sacrosanct Gothic church we find pictures of a rather technical nature, and in the case of the urinal – the main diagnostic instrument of the time – fairly prosaic medical instruments. This combination may seem surprising to modern eyes but to medieval visitors it was completely logical. In earlier times religion and medicine went hand in glove, with Christ himself looked upon as the ultimate healer, often hailed as *Christus Medicus*, who ordered his apostles to spread the Word throughout the world and to heal the sick:

> The apostles left and started telling everyone to turn to God. They forced out many demons and healed a lot of sick people by putting olive oil on them. (Mark 6: 12-13)

The way Cosmas and Damian understood their medical tasks and carried out their profession resembles this calling of Christ. One could say that they behaved like apostles by continuing his healing function. Starting with the legend of Cosmas and Damian, this article will explore the full scope of the medical profession in the Middle Ages and the Renaissance. The brothers were patrons of healing in its various manifestations – surgeons, academically educated doctors, apothecaries, healing saints –, which can be seen in the many pictorial representations to be found in this book.

An antidote for Asclepius

The popularity of the concept of the *Christus Medicus* originated in Late Antiquity and was aimed at shattering the popularity of the pagan healing gods and their sanctuaries as well as the reputation of ancient medical authors. The Church Father Origen, for example, composed a treatise entitled *Contra Celsum* – referring to the popular medical encyclopaedist Celsus. In this text Origen railed against the crowds who visited the temples of Asclepius, seeking their salvation there. Around AD 330, his colleague, the Christian apologist Arnobius, similarly vented his anger on the ancient god of medicine Asclepius by stating that:

> ... he is encased in the shape and compass of the serpent, crawling along the ground after the fashion of worms which spring from mud. He rubs the ground with his chin and breast and drags himself in sinuous coils.

These abusive words seem to refer to the fact that the god's sacred animal was a serpent and that a number of cult legends even describe Asclepius as appearing in the shape of an animal. It is therefore no coincidence that the healing methods of Cosmas and Damian recall the procedures at Asclepian temples, where people spent the night and after such 'incubations' were expected to wake up healed. The story of the transplantation of the black leg, where the patient sleeps through the whole operation, seems inspired by ancient Asclepian procedures and might have been developed to counter the influence of the immensely popular Graeco-Roman god. Looking at the time in which the saints lived, the third century, a period of great Pagan-Christian antagonism – including persecution by the Roman emperor Diocletian – the analogies are logical. There is another element from the *vita* of Cosmas and Damian that refers to the struggle between pagan cults and Christianity and is still of topical interest. The priests at the temples of Asclepius often became very rich from the oblations of grateful patients. Archaeological excavations have found numerous highly valuable votive statuettes of ailing body parts in gold, silver and bronze. Allegedly, Cosmas and Damian operated completely otherwise, treating their patients for free. When Damian broke this rule by accepting three eggs from a woman called Palladia, a scene painted by Fra Angelico on the San Marco Altarpiece, Cosmas became so furious that he requested not to be buried in the same grave as his twin brother. They only made up when God sent a message that Damian was forgiven. The tradition of saints healing for free was especially strong in the Eastern Orthodox Church, where Cosmas and Damian bore the title *anargyroi*, that is, they who decline silver. The discussion about whether or not doctors should accept payment in return for their services continued throughout the Middle Ages. Similar to today, healers were often made out to be greedy. The official designation for a doctor's bill in fact became *honorarium*, meaning that they were expected to do their work primarily for the honour and not for the money.

To circumvent the issue of payment for medical treatment during the Later Middle Ages, many city authorities decided to appoint official town physicians, who in return for a fixed salary would treat poor patients for nothing. To supplement their income the doctors were allowed to treat private patients, who could be charged substantial amounts. The duty to help the poor was part of the system of Acts or Works of Mercy which developed in the Later Middle Ages. Inspired by the works of Christ, they were propagated as acts and practices which believers had to perform to secure the salvation of their souls. They were based on instructions from Jesus, such as that passed on by the evangelist Matthew, 'You shall love your neighbour as yourself', which also implied tending the bodily needs of others, such as 'to feed the hungry, to give drink to the thirsty, to clothe the naked, to harbour the harbourless, to visit the sick, to ransom the captive' and, a later addition, 'to bury the dead'. The system inspired the development of an elaborate system of charity, including hospitals, the distribution of food and clothes, and other forms of poor relief in which all kinds of medical practitioners played a role.

Healing saints

In the wake of Jesus, who during his lifetime had healed several patients and even resurrected people who had died, most saints specialized in certain types of miraculous healing. Often such healing took place via the veneration of miraculous sculptures. Many churches housed such a statue, usually of Mary, and clerical and secular authorities encouraged its cult, helping the local economy to flourish due to the many pilgrims who would flock there. As the church wardens were often expert archivists, documenting the various miracles in 'miracle books', we know that most of them concerned healing. For example, many parents undertook pilgrimages to miraculous statues of Mary because she had revived their child after an apparent drowning, which was more common in times when many could not swim and the majority of canals, ditches, wells and swamps were not fenced. Those who had been cured of blindness, lameness or eyesores also figure frequently in the miracle books. This is not surprising as they were very common complaints at the time.

From the High Middle Ages on, Christians felt a greater need to express their personal devotion and consequently saints became increasingly popular. Their ability to heal was of course also an important reason for their enhanced status. Officially, by the way, they were just intercessors who mediated between the individual and God by bringing the case to His attention. This was thought to be possible because, after their demise, the souls of holy men and women were supposed to rise to heaven, while their mortal remains stayed on earth, often becoming venerated as relics. By touching them the patients made contact with heaven. In cases of recovery many believers were of course convinced that the relic had caused the miracle itself. There are many stories of pilgrims who tried to steal relics, or take a piece of them, or who held a piece of linen or paper against the saintly corpse and thus created a contact relic or *brandeum*, which subsequently was used or sold as an amulet. Such practices were extensively discussed by sixth-century bishop and author Gregory of Tours, who explains his own recovery from dysentery as follows (note the clash of interests between ancient medicine and miracles):

> In the second month after my ordination, when I was at a country place, I suffered from dysentery and high fever and began to be so ill that I altogether despaired of living.

> Everything that I could eat was always vomited before it had been digested and I loathed food, and when my stomach had no more strength as a result of no food the fever was the only thing that gave me strength; I could in no way take anything substantial and strengthening. I had severe pain, too, that darted all through my stomach and went down into my bowels, exhausting me by its pain no less than the fever had done. And when I was in such a condition that no hope of life was left and everything was being made ready for my death and the physician's medicine could do nothing for one whom death had laid claim to, I was in despair and called the chief physician Armentarius and said to him: 'You have used every trick in your profession, you have tried the power of all your remedies, but secular means are of no avail to the perishing. There is only one thing left for me to do. I will show you a great remedy: Let them bring dust from the holy master's tomb [i.e. Saint Martin] and make a potion for me from it. And if this does not cure me, every means of escape is lost.' Then the deacon was sent to the tomb of the holy bishop just mentioned and he brought the sacred dust and put it in water and gave me a drink of it. When I had drunk soon all pain was gone and I received health from the tomb. And the benefit was so immediate that although this happened in the third hour, I became quite well and went to dinner that very day at the sixth hour. (*The Four Books of the Miracles of St. Martin*, II, 1)

There were many relics of Cosmas and Damian in circulation, and those once owned by Gregory ended up in a special cell in the Saint Martin's Church of his home town Tours. There they could be touched and were used to heal his followers. In the tenth century, the skulls of the twin brothers were placed in the Cathedral of Bremen, where at Easter in 1334 they were miraculously rediscovered by Burchard Grelle, Archbishop of Bremen, who personally retrieved the immured relics. Soon afterwards, the Church of Saint Michael in Munich also had a pair on display, which originated in a monastery in Bamberg, while the Convent of the Poor Clares in Madrid also boasted a pair. It is said that Mary of Austria, daughter of Emperor Charles V, donated them to the nuns in 1581.

Some saints specialized in a particular illness. Usually, this specialization had no direct connection to particular cures, but rather with the way their lives had ended in martyrdom, or with the suffering they endured during their lifetimes. In this sense, Cosmas and Damian constitute an exception. They were just exemplary practitioners and generally venerated for that reason rather than their miracle working. One can argue that the later insertion of the miracle of the transplantation into their *vita* was found to be a necessary compensation. Patients seldom invoked their help for direct relief or miracles, as other holy specialists promised more solace. Saint Appollonia, who had been martyred by having her teeth extracted, could be invoked to help toothache; Lucia, whose eyes were gouged out, offered relief for blindness; Cunera, who was killed by strangulation, was called on for sore throats and respiratory difficulties; Sebastian, who died in a hail of arrows, for plague; while the decapitated Saint John was invoked for headaches, mental problems or throat problems. Others had been sufferers themselves, such as Job in the case of leprosy and Roche in the case of plague. They became the patrons of the many specialized hospitals devoted to leprosy and plague which were erected in the Late Middle Ages due to the rise of charity.

Saints, or to be precise aspiring saints, worked most of their miracles after their demise. Their written lives or *vitae* usually recorded these works at the end of the book. Many of these miracles concern marvellous recoveries resulting from the invocation of such a saint. In the canonization processes that were necessary to sanctify these men and women, these wonders in particular were used as corroboration. Quite paradoxically to modern eyes, medical doctors were asked to examine the recovery of the patients concerned. Using all their medical expertise, they were to judge and categorize the ailment, the behaviour of and therapies used on the patient and ultimately the manner by which they were cured. In cases where a medical doctor came to the conclusion that the recovery could be explained by natural causes, the canonization process came to a halt. A recovery was only deemed miraculous when it could not be accounted for medically and thus could be attributed to divine intervention.

This way of determining miracles was also the case for the many physical sufferings that holy men and women underwent themselves. The fourteenth-century saint Catherine of Siena, for example, fasted for years, which according to her *vita* was possible because her constitution was sustained by one consecrated host. Modern authors of course have asserted that she might have been anorexic, but contemporary physicians classified her ability to live without food as miraculous.

Many holy men and women were thought to suffer from heart problems due to the belief that their soul, which was situated in the heart, was in continuous connection with the Holy Spirit. The Umbrian prioress, Chiara da Montefalco (*c.*1300), is a perfect example of a saintly heart patient. She claimed to have shared Christ's burden by helping him to bear the Cross. The bond between her and Christ was so close that objects related to Christ's Passion materialized in her heart. After her death the local surgeon and a couple of nuns, probably country girls who knew how to slaughter animals, cut her heart open and found the incarnated objects within. They jointly prepared the corpse, which, together with the heart and the nails, is still on display in the Umbrian town of Montefalco. In 1985 medical professors examined the heart one last time and found it had been miraculously healthy despite the saint's tremendous suffering.

The formation of Western European medicine

The concepts used and the procedures that were followed within medicine were not a medieval invention but stemmed from Antiquity. Most of the important ancient medical writers were translated and commented upon by Arab medical writers in the Early Middle Ages. From the eleventh century onwards, medical treatises became available in Latin thanks to the efforts of translators in Toledo and Southern Italy, where the Arab, Greek and Western European cultures stood in close contact.

Constantinus Africanus (*c.*1087), a monk from the famous Benedictine monastery of Cassino – but as his name suggests from Muslim origin – translated many Arab treatises that were based on the Greek physicians Hippocrates and Galen. These works constituted the core curriculum of the medical school of Salerno, often regarded as the first medical faculty in Europe, and soon found acceptance elsewhere. Masters were instructing their students using such texts, as well as practical medicine. Still well known today is the *Regimen Salernitatum*, which contained the basic dietary guidelines for the preservation or recovery of health in the Middle Ages. Thousands of manuscripts of this work, which are often beautifully illustrated, are still in existence. This also applies to the gynaecological treatises by Trota (or Trotula), who was a female practitioner and author in Salerno in the twelfth century. Summaries of her work were composed and translated into the vernacular for the instruction of midwives in the fourteenth and fifteenth centuries.

The study of medicine concentrated on the organization and functioning of the healthy human body. In this, medical students followed the Persian physician and philosopher Ibn Sīnā (*c.*980-1037), better known under his Latinized name Avicenna, whose famous *Canon Medicinae* had to be learned by heart when commencing medical instruction at university. The handbook opens with the following definition of medicine:

> Medicine is the science by which the dispositions of the human body are known so that whatever is necessary is removed or healed by it, in order that health should be preserved or, if absent, recovered.

This meant that medical knowledge was mainly physiological and anatomical. It aimed at understanding the functioning of the healthy human body, with pathology secondary. As this was unsatisfactory for many healers, the Later Middle Ages saw the production of many practical handbooks which listed the diseases of the body parts and their remedies *a capite ad calcem*, from head to toe.

The point of departure for medicine was the preservation of an equilibrium in terms of *complexio* or, in Greek, *crasis*, translated as 'temperament'. *Complexio* refers to a well-balanced combination of the elementary qualities of hot, cold, dry and wet within a human body. The theory was introduced by Hippocrates and Galen but elaborated into a system by Avicenna. It functioned as a system of explanation, whereby disease was viewed as occurring due to an imbalance in the qualities, with the balance to be restored by therapy or medication. As every human being had his or her own innate temperament, it was the organizing principle of each human. Reasoning based on temperament permeated everything, including human body parts. The heart, for example, was hot, while the brain was cold. The system can be deemed holistic since mind and matter were seen as directly interconnected. The temperament determined all human characteristics, including the psychological, something which is still echoed in the modern use of the word temperament in relation to designations such as 'choleric' and 'melancholic'. The individual *complexio* was thought to be influenced by external circumstances, such as the environment in which one lived, the time of year, sex, age and of course exercise and nutrition. Heat and moisture were seen as positive, but over time they would unfortunately be replaced by the coldness and dryness of advanced years.

To understand the concept of *complexio*, doctors and philosophers also used the system of the four elements and the four humours. These ideas can be traced back to Greek authors such as Hippocrates, Aristotle and of course Galen, but again they were worked into a system by Avicenna. The latter's *Canon* laid down the standard set of four humours: blood, phlegm, yellow bile and black bile, which were seen as crucial for the physiological functioning of the human body. Some authors connected the quantity of bodily fluids to the life span of the person. When all bodily fluids had been used or dried up, death followed.

During the Middle Ages and the Renaissance diagnosis and therapy were very much determined by the theory of the humours. Treatment revolved around removing excess and supplementing shortage. The popular practices of bloodletting, the setting of leeches, bathing or sweating were all based on assumptions about the roles of humours, elements and qualities. Although an equilibrium of humours was preferable, one humour was considered to be more precious than the others, with bloody types being regarded as the best kind of human being, especially when they were in their prime. Here we meet an interrelation of religion and medicine, since Jesus, who died at 33 and bled profusely, was presented as one of the prototypes of the favourable bloody temperament.

The same mixture of religious and medical concepts is found in the discussion on the hierarchy of human body parts. Aristotle had asserted that the human heart was the most important, as its beat announced the coming into being of new life, while its cessation meant death. Galen, however, taught the theory of the three principal members – brain, heart and liver – each governing its own group of organs and functions. Although all three of these had a soul, for Galen, the brain was the most important and was concerned with rationality. In the twelfth century, Aristotle's natural philosophical works were rediscovered and translated into Latin at the same time that religion intensified and increasingly acquired a more physical dimension. Despite the fact that many medical doctors acknowledged that the brain had a directing function via the nerves, the heart maintained its prime position. It was in the warm heart that the Holy Spirit ignited religious fervour. Many saints were literally ablaze with holy fire, which in the case of Chiara da Montefalco and Catherine of Siena, resulted in major heart diseases. Catherine allegedly exchanged her heart for that of Christ, which is also shown dripping with blood in many altarpieces.

Anatomical knowledge

In the twelfth and thirteenth centuries, noblemen often went on crusades and sometimes died far from home. This meant that, in order to guarantee that their corpse could be buried in the royal vault, a dissection was necessary. This happened to the remains of King Louis XI of France, who died near Tunis on 25 August 1270 on his second crusade. According to a tradition known as *Mos Teutonicus*, his flesh was boiled from his body so that the bones could be transported home. The skeleton was taken to the French royal necropolis at Saint Denis. Most of his entrails were buried immediately on the spot; however, his heart was placed in an urn and taken to the basilica of Monreale at Palermo, where it still remains. The burying of royal body parts separately became a tradition, with the body of a French king usually being taken to Saint Denis and his heart being interred in the chapel of the royal palace in Paris. Other emperors, kings and popes, and soon also other members of the higher nobility, followed the custom.

This habit may seem crude but it was simply practical. Often the remains of highly placed persons were the centre of elaborate funerary rituals, including lying in state for days, if not weeks, in the important cities of their realm. In such cases a post-mortem examination was also carried out, usually by surgeons working at court and under the supervision of the court physicians. Lying in state was not the only reason for dissection. In cases where a king or pope had died under suspicious circumstances, family and friends often wanted to know why and requested what we would call a forensic examination. In such cases the surgeons and medical doctors closely recorded the anatomical details they discerned and used these in their teaching and practices.

Despite what is often believed, the Church did not forbid anatomical examination. On the contrary, anatomical knowledge was crucial for the manufacturing of relics, and medical knowledge was a *sine qua non* in canonization processes. From the thirteenth century onwards, as the medical faculties of the papally approved universities developed, anatomy became a regular part of the curriculum. Witnessing an autopsy was an essential requirement for medical students wishing to graduate. It is nevertheless true that they were a rare phenomenon, for which there were various reasons, but these do not include a clerical ban. The first concerns the general taboo around death and the handling of cadavers, which prevails in every society. In Greek and Roman society the abhorrence of touching human cadavers had been so strong that almost no anatomical research was carried out. Galen's anatomical knowledge was based on the dissection of dogs, monkeys and pigs or stemmed from his practice as a physician to the gladiators of Rome. As medieval medicine generally followed ancient examples, doctors at the time were not encouraged to undertake independent anatomical research. At public anatomical lessons, the professor would read out texts by Galen or Avicenna while a surgeon dissected the body and an assistant pointed out the organs under discussion. The whole procedure functioned mainly as a live illustration of an anatomical text. Another reason for the infrequency of autopsies was the inadequate climatic conditions for a prolonged examination. This was especially an issue in Italy, which nevertheless offered the best medical education and on this basis attracted the majority of Northern European students. Most public autopsies, however, only took place in the winter. Quite often they were part of the festivities of the Carnival season. Apart from the fact that the weather was cold, it was found to be an appropriate time to confront death. The dissection of a cadaver was a macabre piece of theatre, enhanced by the public display of dressed-up skeletons, hour glasses and other symbols of the fragility of human life that would prominently figure during Lent. Of course these rituals also pointed to the soon to be remembered death of Christ on the Cross.

Medical hierarchy

The division of roles during a dissection indicates the existence of a certain hierarchy within the medical profession, although we should not take that division of roles too strictly. In general, a university-educated medical doctor stuck to his books, diagnosed by inspecting the patient's urine or feeling the pulse and then prescribed a therapy, usually executed by a surgeon or an apothecary. The former treated wounds or let blood and would have served a long apprenticeship with a master and certainly would not be illiterate. Several surgeons' manuals have survived from the Middle Ages because they were rapidly put into print at the end of the fifteenth century, a testament to both their popularity and the literacy of their users. They were usually adaptations in the vernacular of Lanfranc of Milano's *Chirurgia Magna* (1296) or Guy de Chauliac's *Inventarium sive collectorium in parte chirurgicali medicinae* (1363). Chauliac's bulky treatise covers many anatomically related topics and techniques and is hailed as the greatest surgical encyclopaedia of the Middle Ages. The text discusses the treatment of wounds, ulcers, fractures, dislocations, the extraction of teeth and a variety of other conditions and diseases, within a broad framework of medical (physiological and pathological) learning. De Chauliac also maintained strong ties with the Church. As well as working as a surgeon in Lyon and lecturing at the University of Poitiers, he worked at the Papal Court at Avignon serving as personal physician to several popes. Some scholars believe that he wrote his treatise with his patients at the Papal Court in mind.

While medical science is an invention of Antiquity, the rise of a medical profession constituted by diverse recognized practitioners with specific qualifications is a product of the Middle Ages. Initiated in the twelfth century by the rulers of Southern Italy such as Roger of Sicily and his grandson Emperor Frederick II, procedures for licensing began. The latter introduced licensing examinations and entrusted these to masters trained in Salerno. By the Late Middle Ages this resulted in an extensive system which could attest to and evaluate the competence of all types of medical practitioners, deeming their activities legitimate or illegitimate. The last category were scorned as being 'empirical' or even 'quacks', referring to the fact that their expertise was merely based on experience and could not be considered expertise built on learning. The term 'quack' is probably derived from an archaic word of Dutch origin, 'quacksalver', meaning 'seller of salve', referring to those who sold popular ointments at the markets, apparently shouting in a loud voice. Another possible derivation is 'quicksilver', as they were mercury-based ointments administered to fight skin diseases.

Encouraged by the authorities, practitioners in many towns formed organizations that regulated the admission of new members through examinations. Some of them, usually those who had received their training at a university, obtained the right to approve other medical healers. In thirteenth-century Italy, craft guilds relating to medical practice were also to be found. In 1293, the *medici*, grocers and apothecaries of Florence formed a guild, from which the academic medical doctors broke away in 1392 to start their own circle. In many cases, Cosmas and Damian functioned as the patrons of these guilds, symbolizing the members' exemplary professional conduct. By the end of the Middle Ages, skilled surgeons also formed their own organizations to emphasize the fact that they were far better than the uneducated barber-surgeons who based their actions solely on practical experience. At the same time, most cities appointed civic medical and surgical practitioners who treated the poor, but also had a legal function in examining the victims of murders or violent attacks, participants in fights and other illegal violence. Usually the academics were in charge of other practitioners, including apothecaries and midwives, to whom they sometimes gave crash courses in basic botany or anatomy.

Cosmas and Damian are therefore connected to the growing organization of the medical profession and also to an increase in confidence and consciousness of the diversity of the field by its members. Some of their depictions were commissioned by medical guilds, others by confraternities directed towards helping the sick or by hospital authorities. The way they are portrayed often gives us a glimpse of their newly acquired confidence. From the Greek doctor-slaves of Roman Antiquity, doctors had become proud, often wealthy upper-class citizens. That the de facto rulers of Florence, the Medici family, did not conceal their medical origin but cherished Cosmas and Damian is apparent from the fact that they erected statues of the brothers in prominent places. Most depictions, but not all, reflect the hierarchy which had arisen within the medical profession. Cosmas represents the university-trained doctor, standing to one side and often shown with a heavy volume and clad in the long robe of the scholar. Damian wears the short robe of the craftsman – the surgeon – and is shown with a surgical knife and the instruments for treating wounds – a spatula and a jar of ointment. However, several pictures in this book show that hierarchical differences were not always as great, with the brothers depicted in more or less the same manner and seeming to proceed in mutual agreement. In many cities, medical doctors and surgeons were still part of the same guilds and sometimes surgeons went to universities at an advanced age to become medical doctors. The anatomical revolution of the sixteenth century, when academic doctors learned to perform their own dissections, being taught by experienced surgeons, shows that working together, combining text-based learning with anatomical research and clinical practice, was the right track for the advance of medical science. In this, the inseparable twin brothers Cosmas and Damian had also shown the way by jointly amputating a leg and replacing it with a healthy black specimen.

Literature

Angenendt, A. 1997. *Heiligen und Reliquien. Die Geschichte ihres Kultes vom frühen Christentum bis zur Gegenwart,* Munich.

Huisman, F.G. 1998. 'Human frailty versus God's omnipotence: the meaning of the Miracle of the Black Leg', in Kees W. Zimmerman, ed., *One Leg in the Grave. The Miracle of the Transplantation of the Black Leg by the Saints Cosmas and Damian*, Maarssen 43-60.

Siraisi, N.G. 1990. *Medieval & Early Renaissance Medicine. An Introduction to Knowledge and Practice,* Chicago.

Biller, P., Ziegler, J. 2001. *Religion and Medicine in the Middle Ages*, Woodbridge.

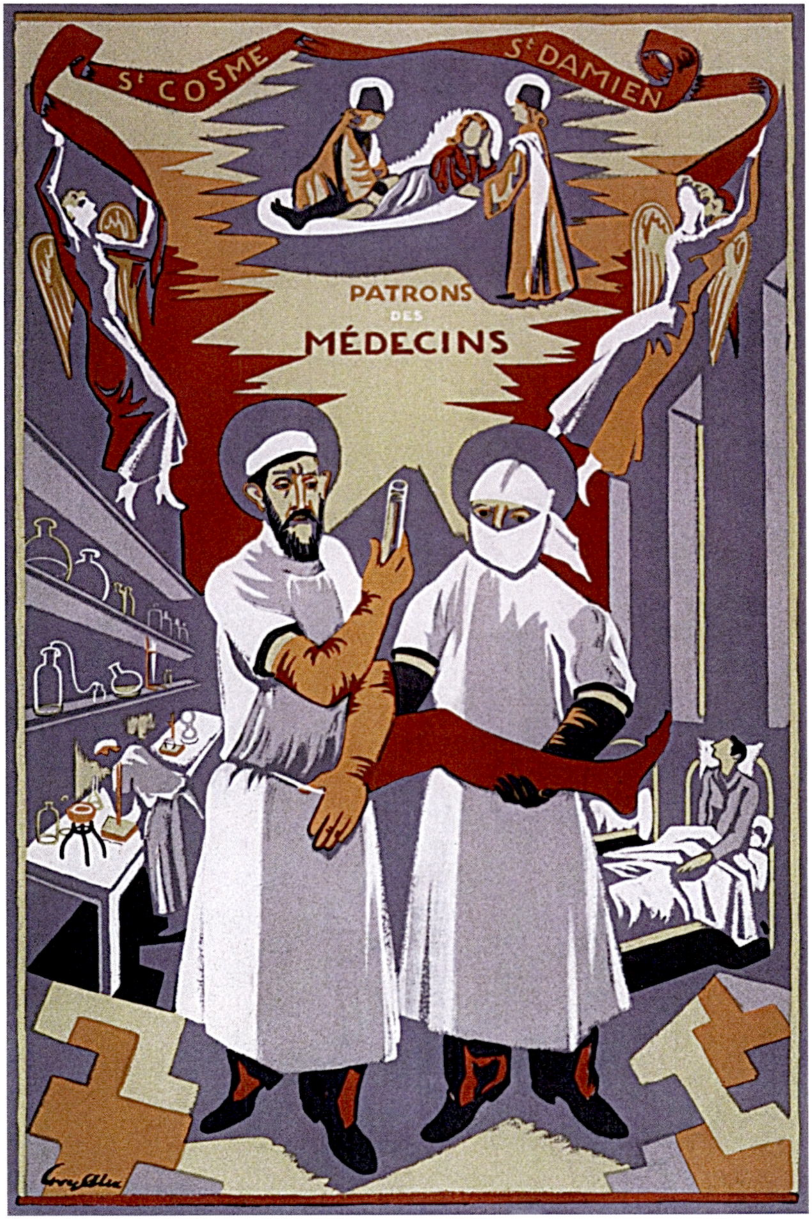

62. **Yves Alix** (1890-1969), *woodcut*. Bibliothèque Nationale, Paris (France).

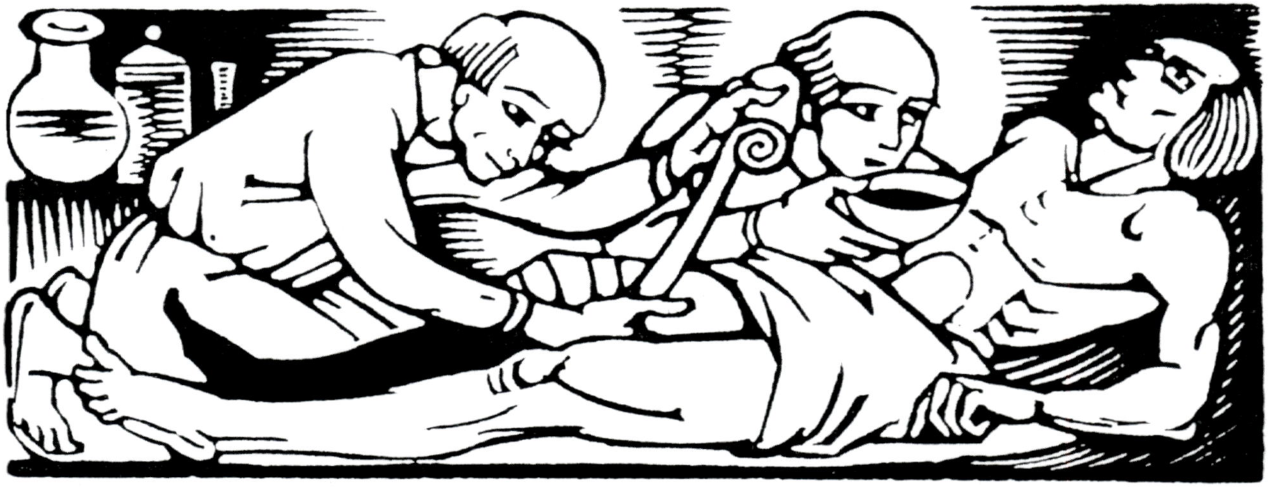

63. **Jean-André Chieze** (1898-1975), *woodcut print*. Musée des Arts et Traditions Populaires, Paris (France).

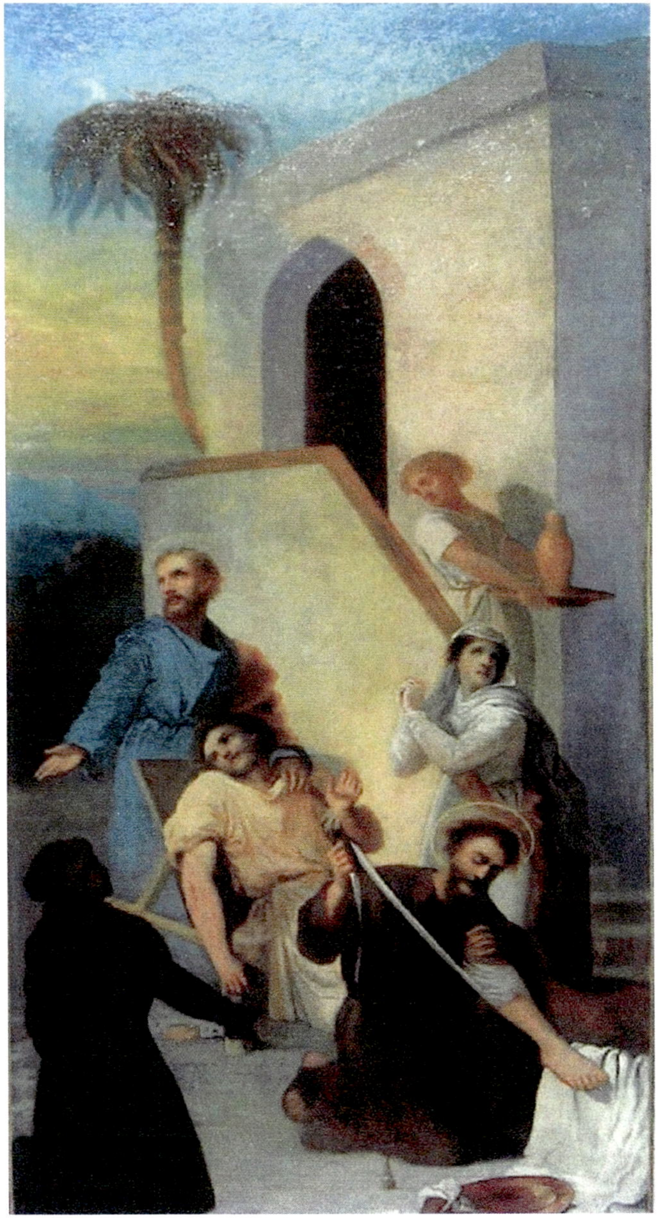

64. **Anonymous,** *painting,* 19th century. Notredame, Montesson (France).

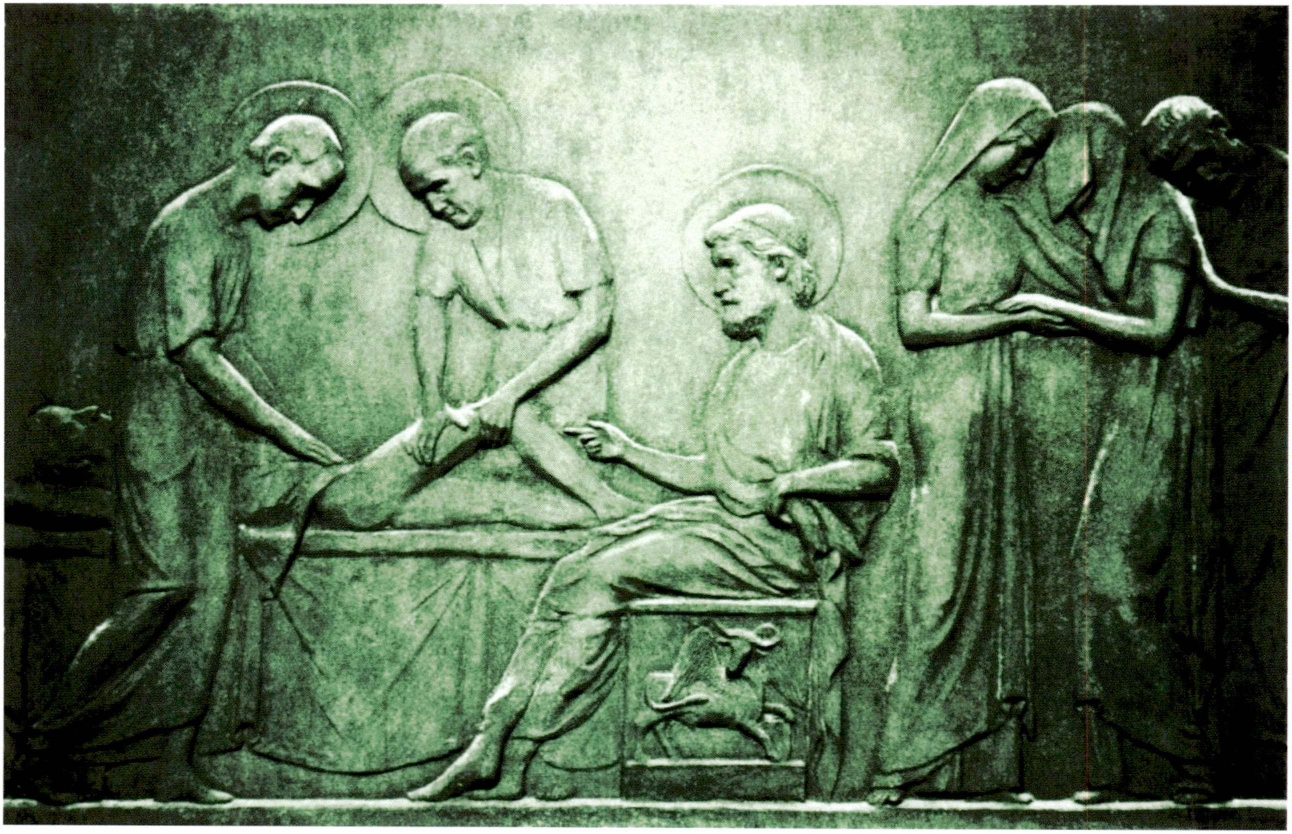

65. **Charles Villandre,** *copper relief,* 1933. Chapelle de l' hôpital Saint Joseph, Paris (France).

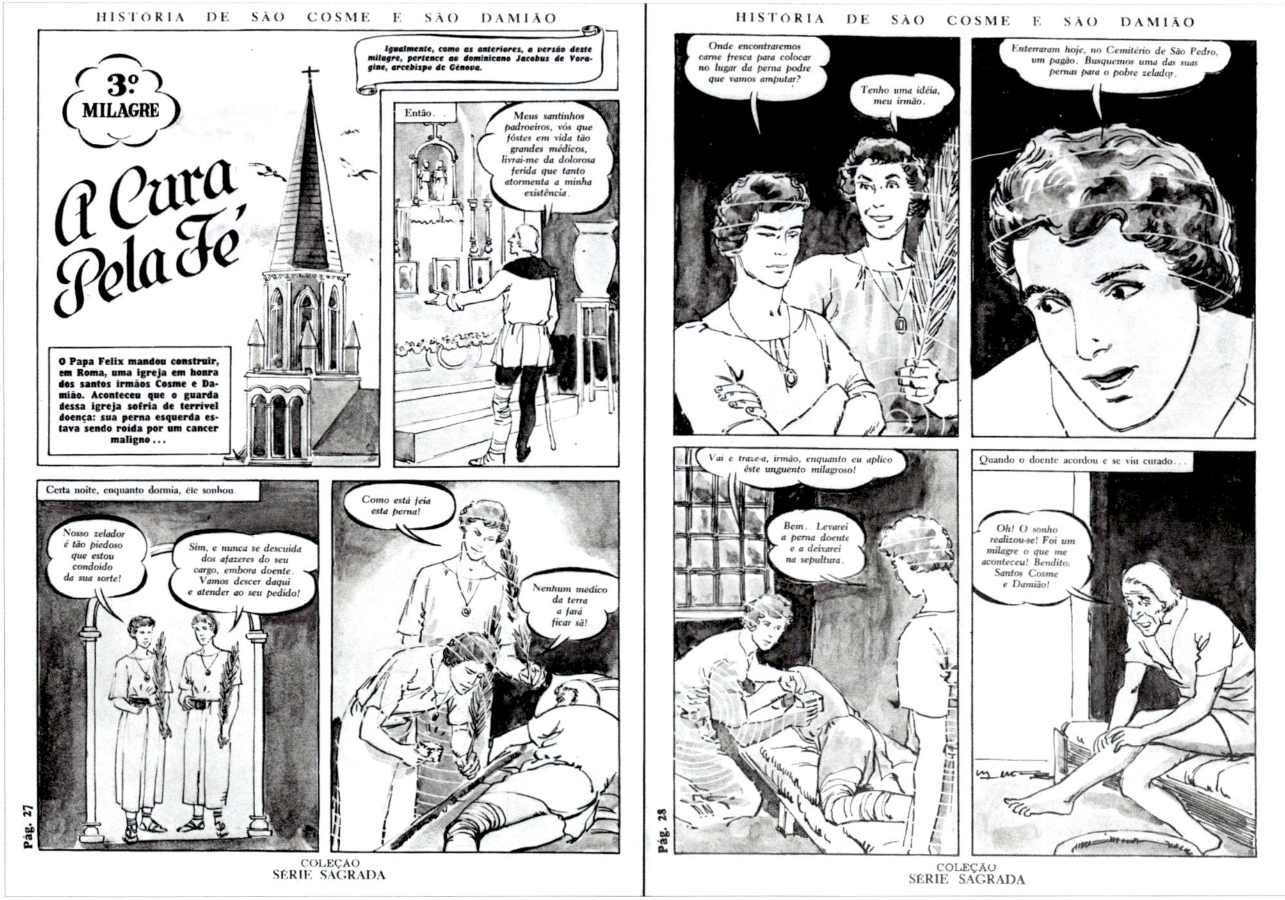
HISTÓRIA DE SÃO COSME E SÃO DAMIÃO
Igualmente, como as anteriores, a versão deste milagre, pertence ao dominicano Jacobus de Voragine, arcebispo de Gênova.
3º MILAGRE
A Cura Pela Fé
O Papa Felix mandou construir, em Roma, uma igreja em honra dos santos irmãos Cosme e Damião. Aconteceu que o guarda dessa igreja sofria de terrível doença: sua perna esquerda estava sendo roída por um cancer maligno . . .
Então. . .
Meus santinhos padroeiros, vós que fôstes em vida tão grandes médicos, livrai-me da dolorosa ferida que tanto atormenta a minha existência.
Certa noite, enquanto dormia, êle sonhou.
Nosso zelador é tão piedoso que estou condoído da sua sorte!
Sim, e nunca se descuida dos afazeres do seu cargo, embora doente. Vamos descer daqui e atender ao seu pedido!
Como está feia esta perna!
Nenhum médico da terra a fará ficar sã!
Pág. 27
COLEÇÃO SÉRIE SAGRADA
HISTÓRIA DE SÃO COSME E SÃO DAMIÃO
Onde encontraremos carne fresca para colocar no lugar da perna podre que vamos amputar?
Tenho uma idéia, meu irmão.
Enterraram hoje, no Cemitério de São Pedro, um pagão. Busquemos uma das suas pernas para o pobre zelador.
Vai e traze-a, irmão, enquanto eu aplico êste unguento milagroso!
Bem. Levarei a perna doente e a deixarei na sepultura.
Quando o doente acordou e se viu curado. . .
Oh! O sonho realizou-se! Foi um milagre o que me aconteceu! Benditos Santos Cosme e Damião!
Pág. 28
COLEÇÃO SÉRIE SAGRADA

66. **Anonymous,** *book,* Série Sagrada: História de São Cosme e São Damião 1954. Brasil.

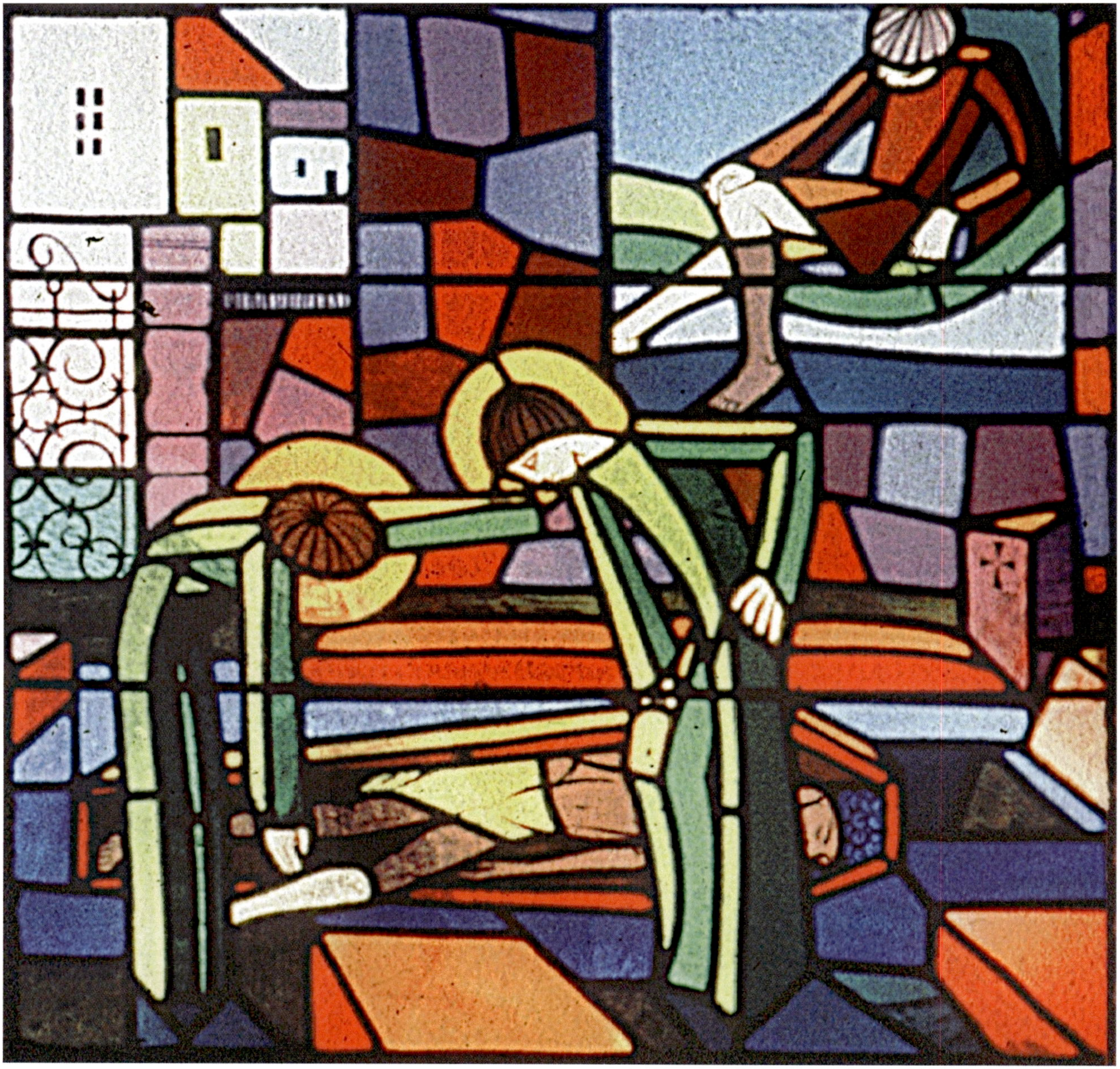

67. **Abbé Louis Ribes,** *stained glass,* 1962. Église Saint Côme et Saint Damien, Caluire (France).

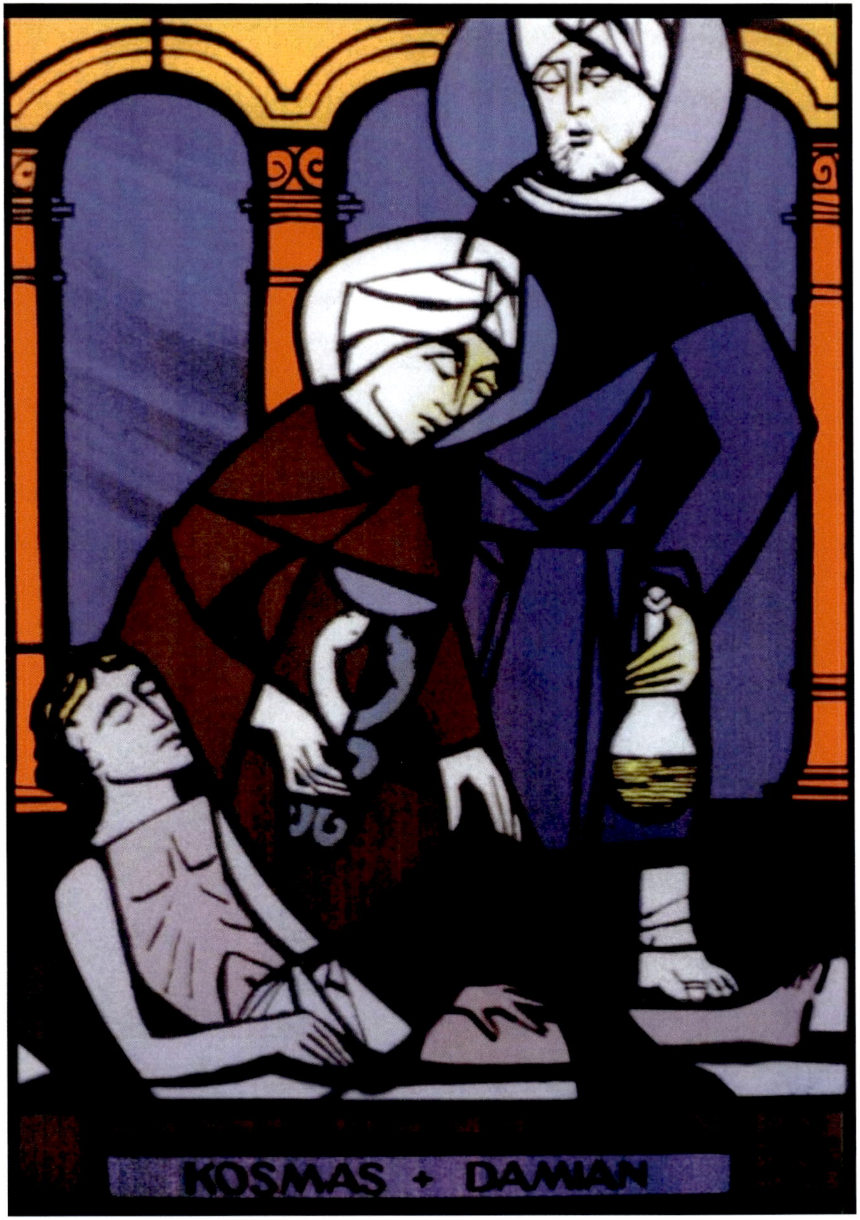

68. **Christoph Stooss,** *stained glass*, 1922. Ärztegesellschaft des Kantons Luzern, Luzern (Switserland).

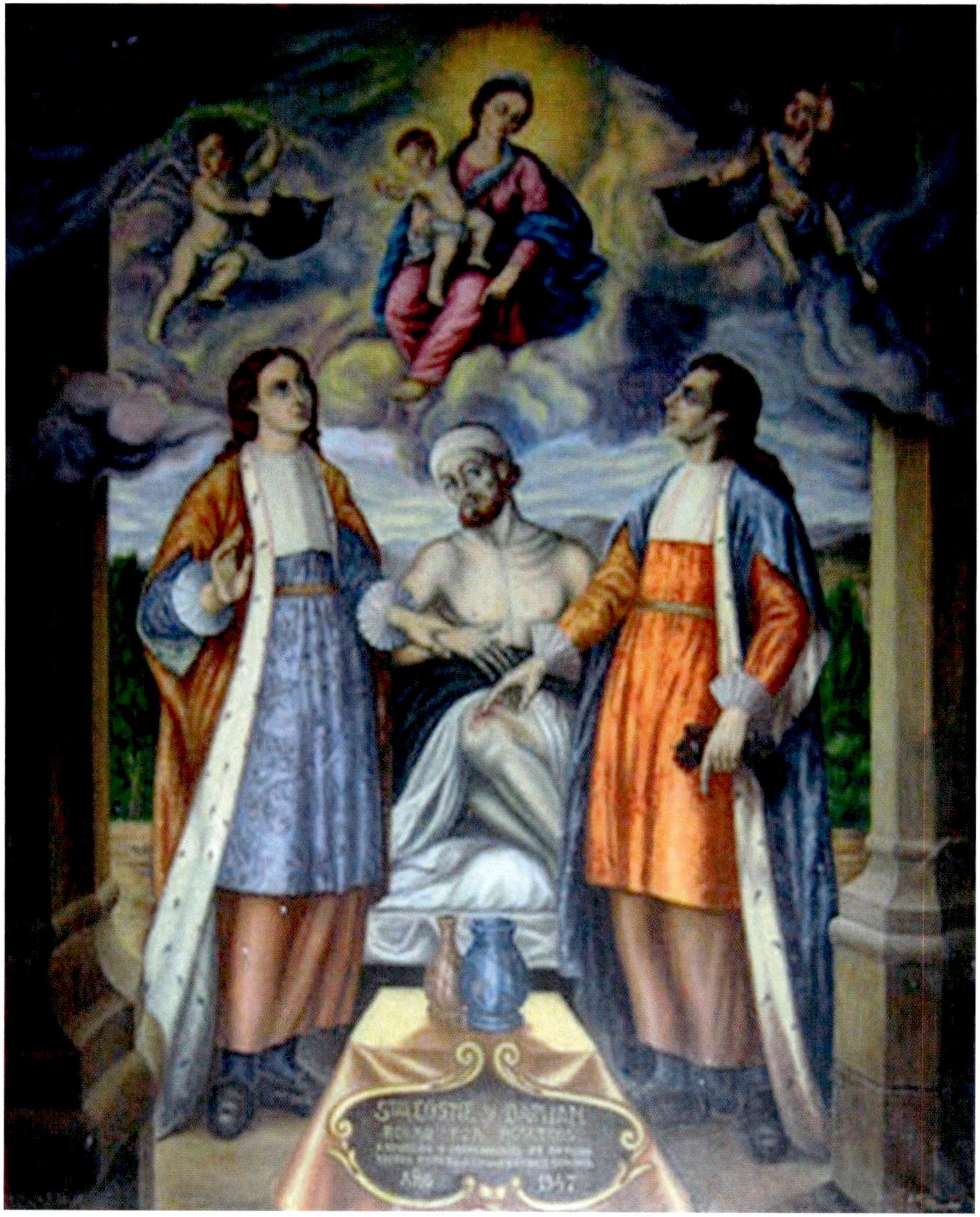

69. **E.Rojo,** *painting*, 1947. Iglesia de Santiago, Lorca (Spain).

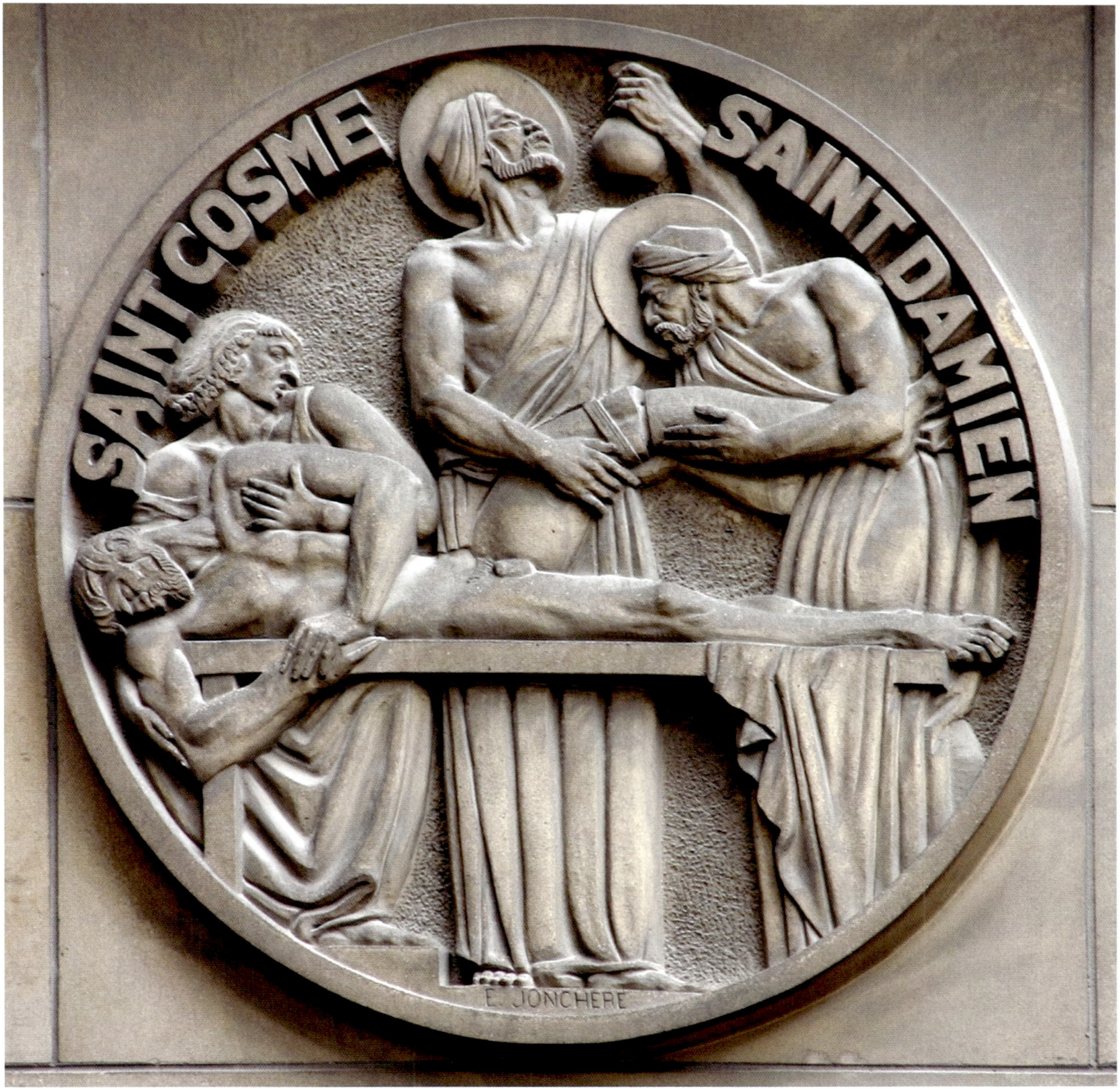

70. **Évariste Jonchère** (1892–1956), *sculpture in sandstone,* 1953. Nouvelle faculté de medicine, Paris (France).

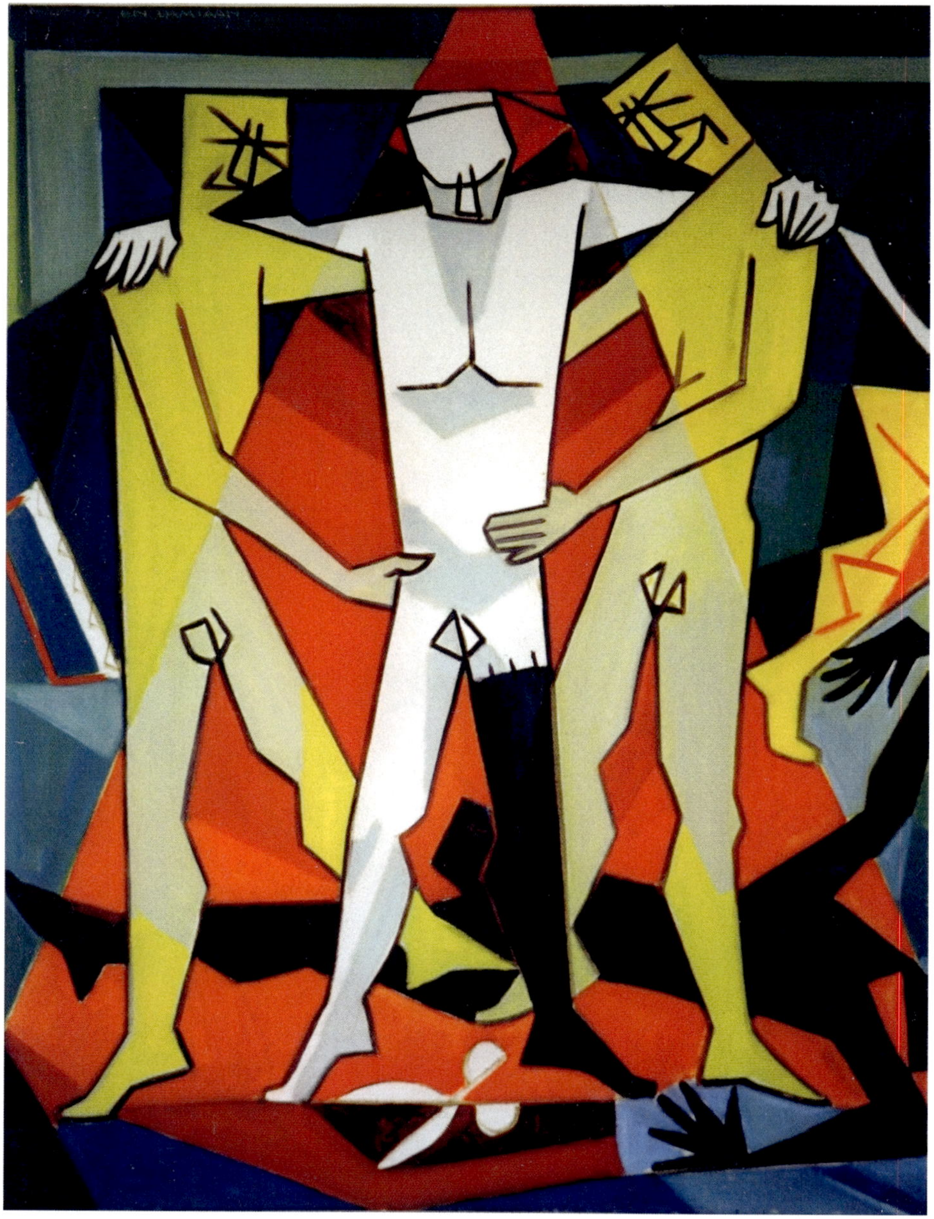

71. **Siep van de Berg** (1913-1998), *painting*, 1955. Private collection, Groningen (the Netherlands).

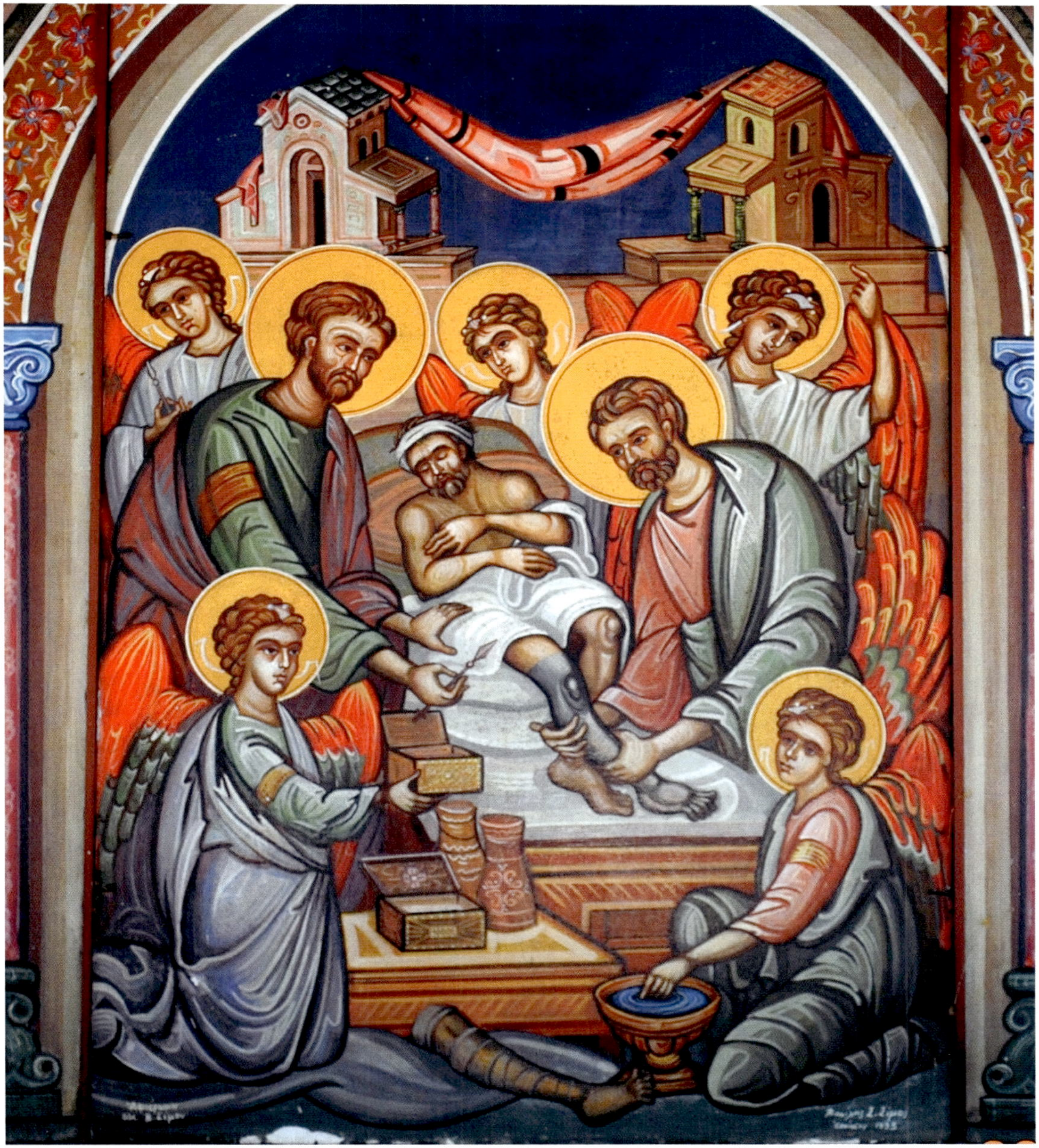

72. Vasilios S. Simons, *icon,* 1993. Μονή Αγάθωνος (Monastero Agathonos), Fthiotida (Greece).

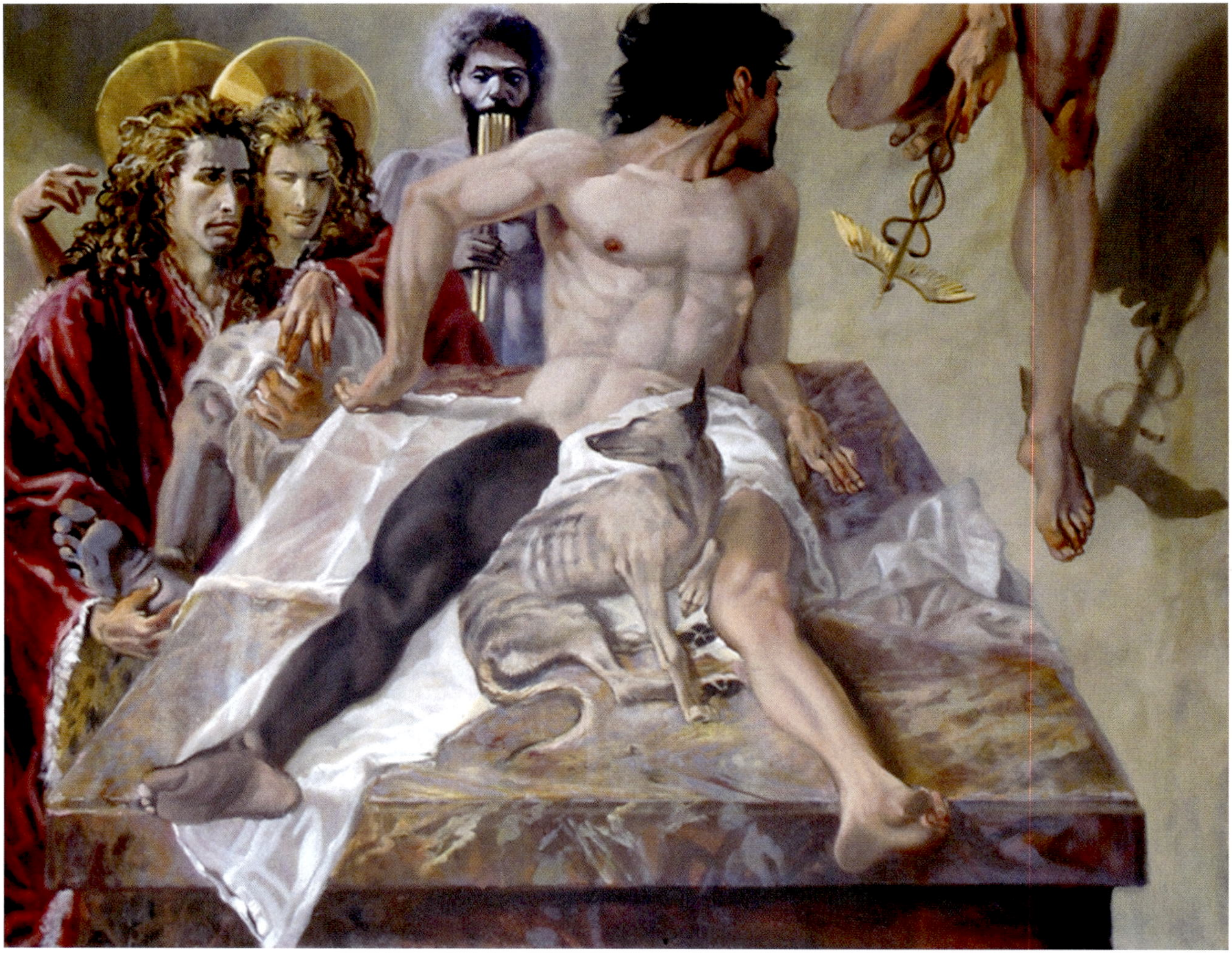

73. **André Durand** (born 1947), *painting*, 1997. Private collection. (V.S.).

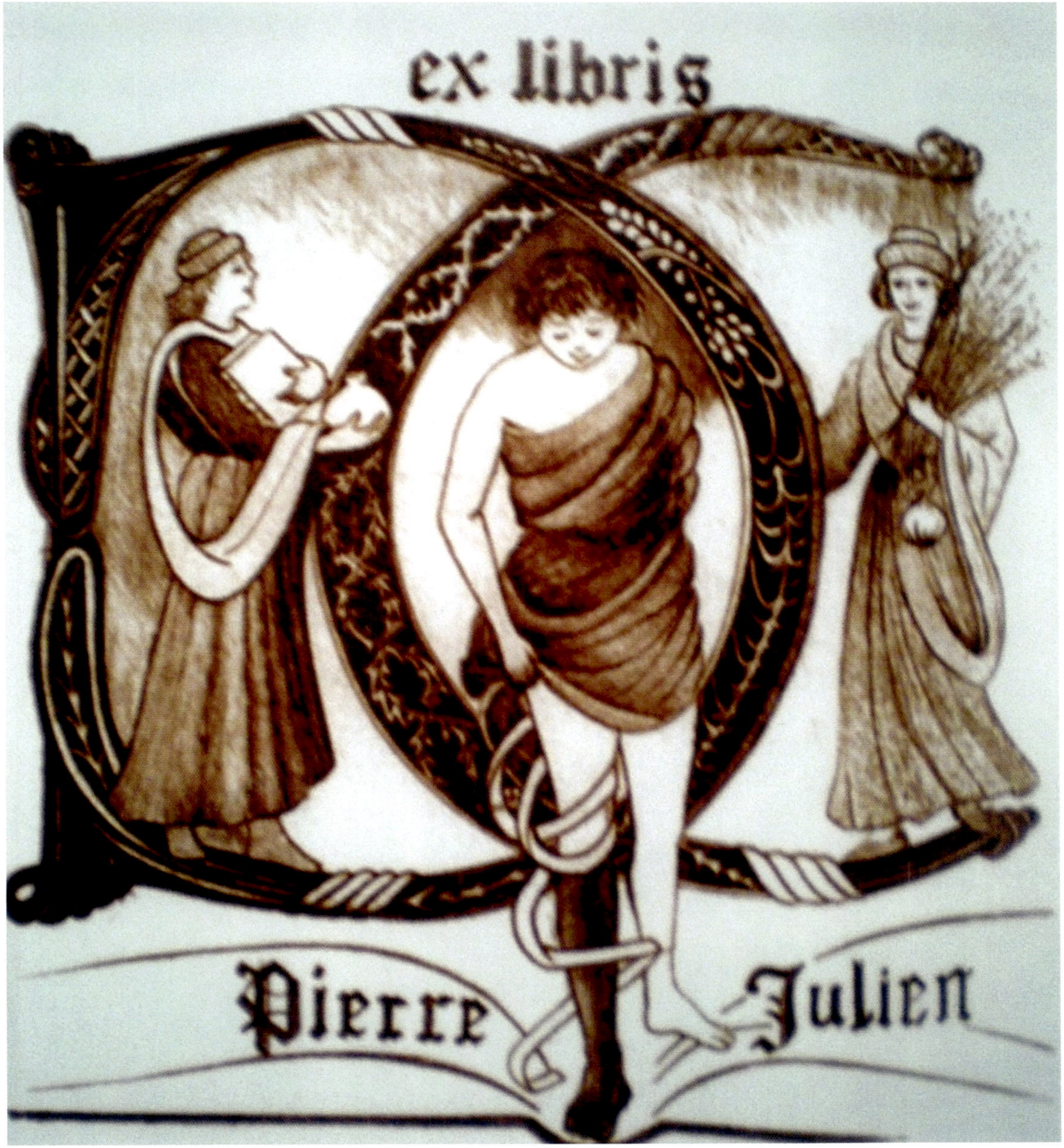

74. **Hélène Nué,** *Ex Libris Pierre Julien,* 2000. Paris (France).

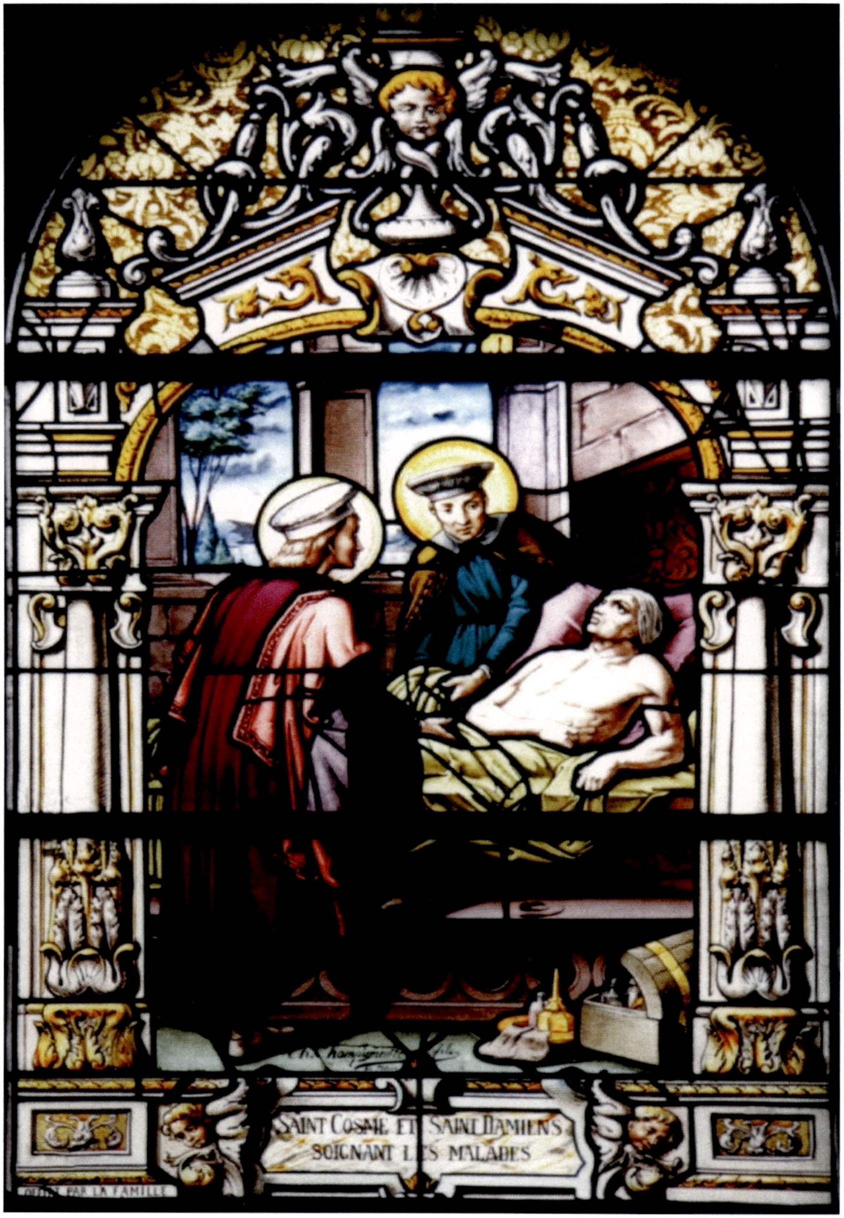
SAINT COSME ET SAINT DAMIENS
SOIGNANT LES MALADES
PAR LA FAMILLE

75. Ch. Lampignuitte, *stained glass,* based on Peselino's painting, 20th century. Églises Saint Côme et Saint Damien, Villebon s. Yvette, (France).

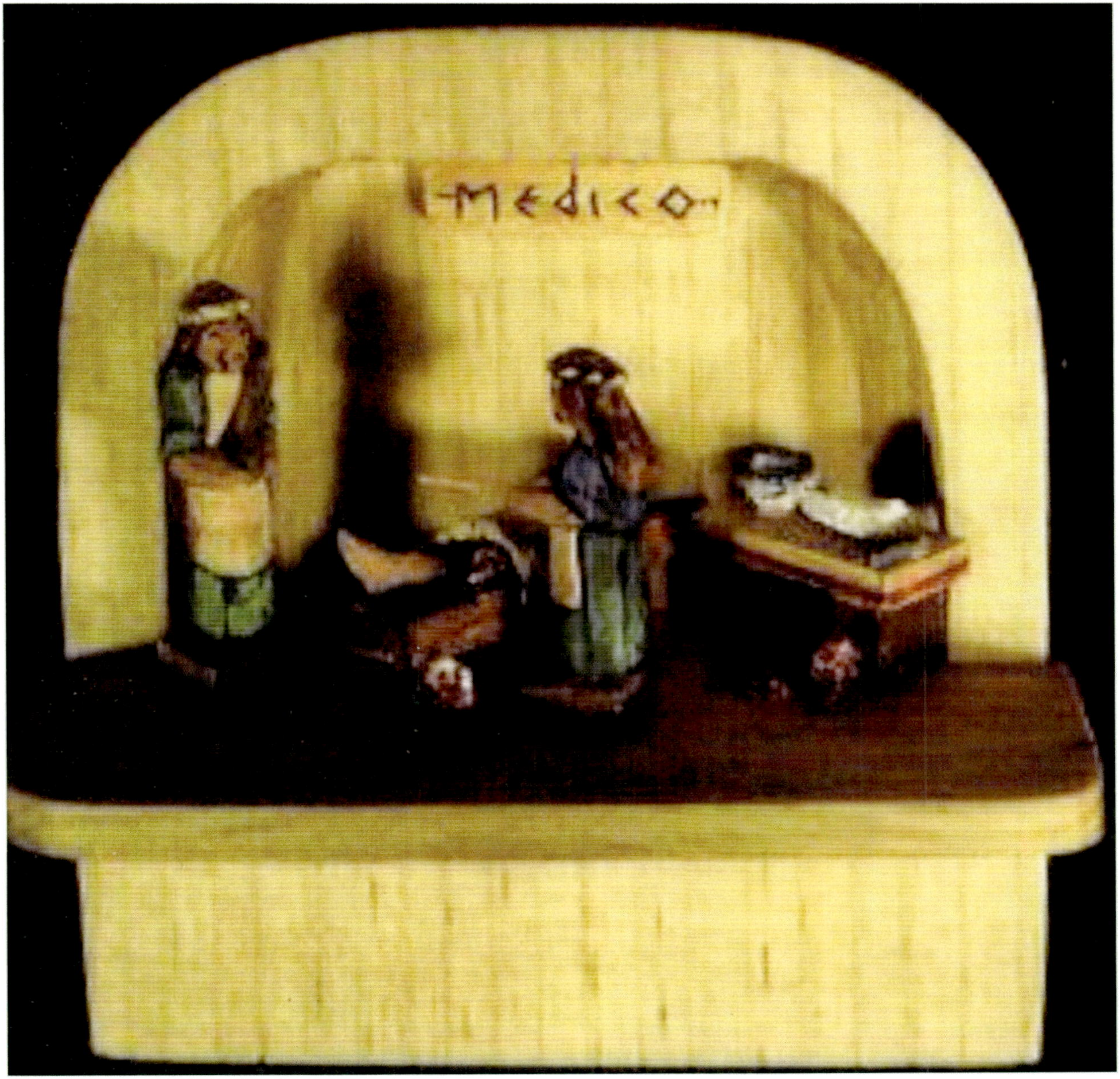

76. **Tomasita J. Rodriguez,** *inlaid nichos (pine wood),* IN008, 20th century. Private collection, Santa Fe (U.S.A.).

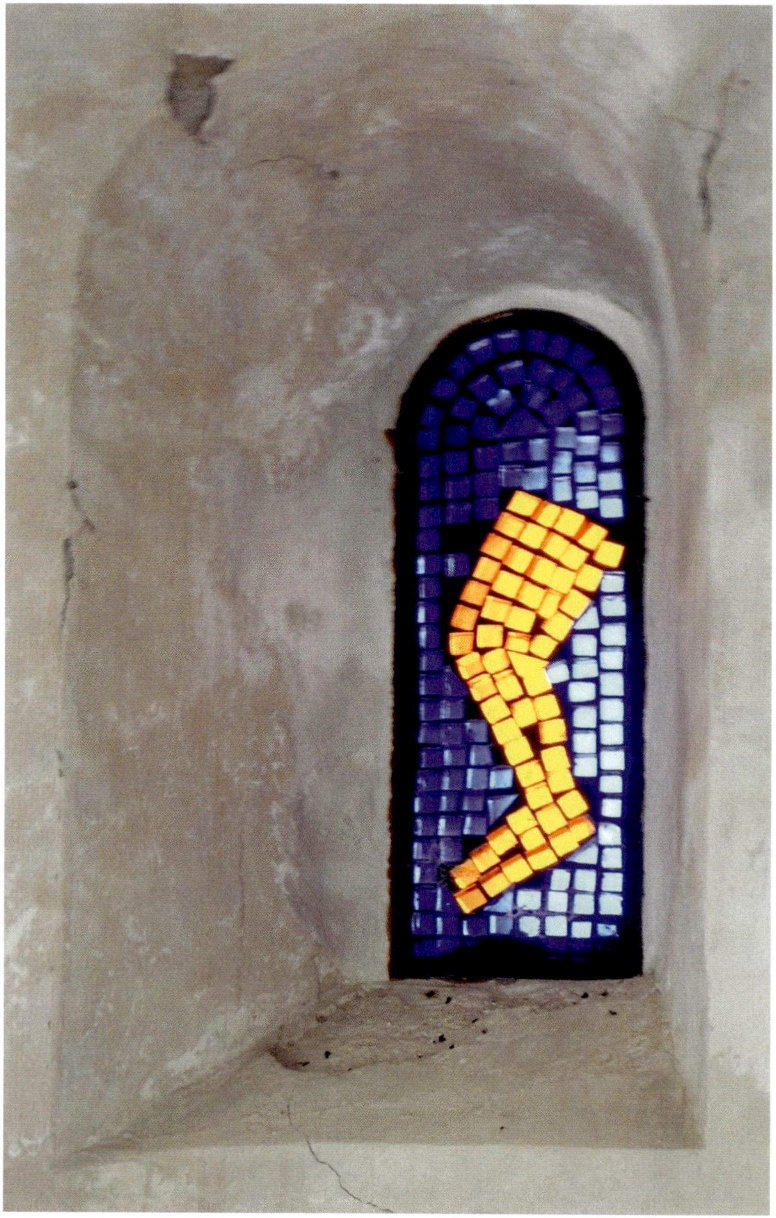

77. **Anonymous,** *stained glass,* 20th century. Chapelle St. Côme, Gigondas (France).

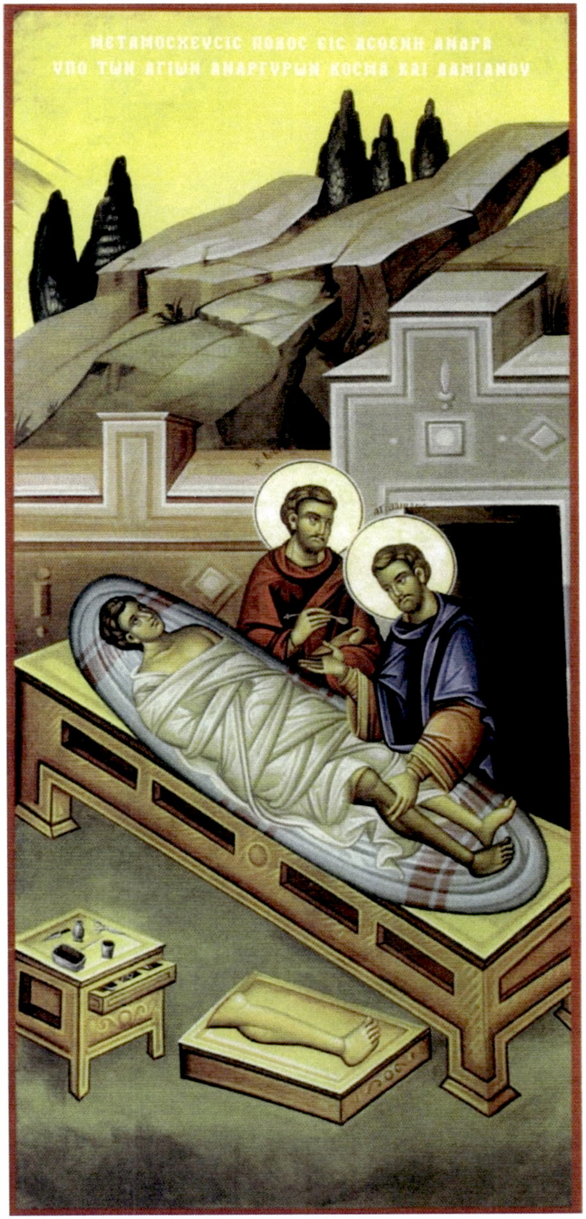

78. **Stravos Gospodinis,** *wallpainting*, 2000. εκκλησία Κοσμάς και Δαμιανός (Church of Cosmas and Damian), Veria (Greece).

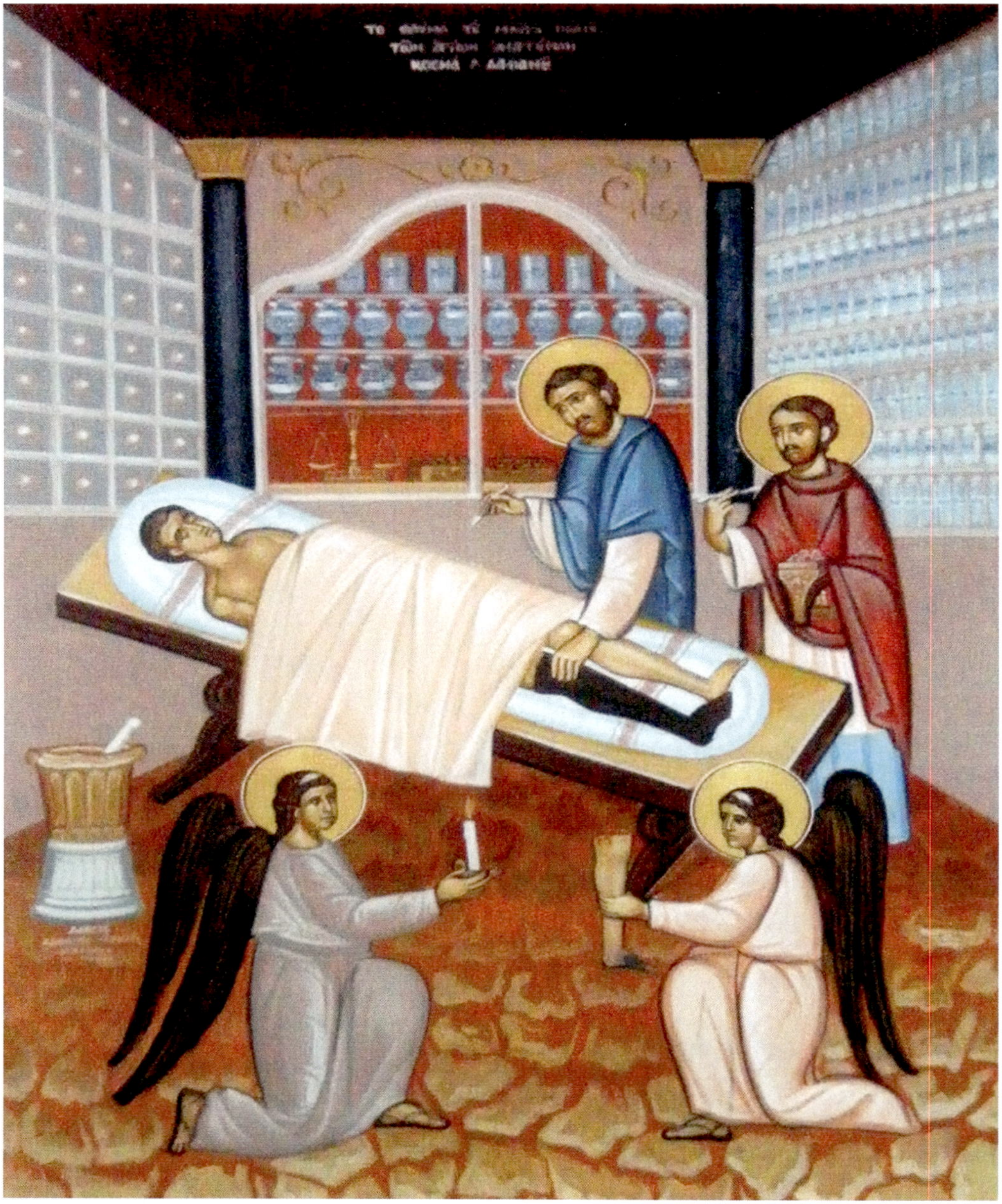

79. Francos Nicolaos, *painting,* 2010. Private collection, Chios (Greece).

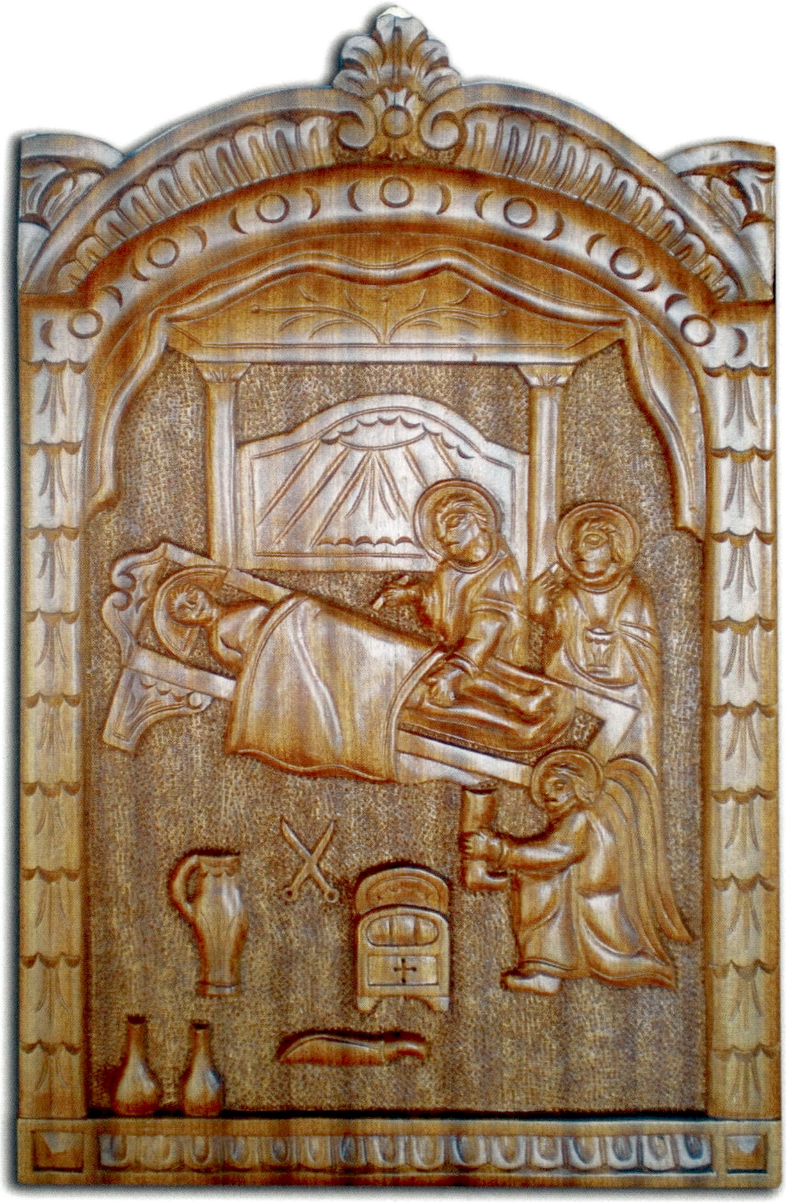

80. **Mastorakis Ioannis,** *woodcarving,* 2011. Private collection, Chios (Greece).

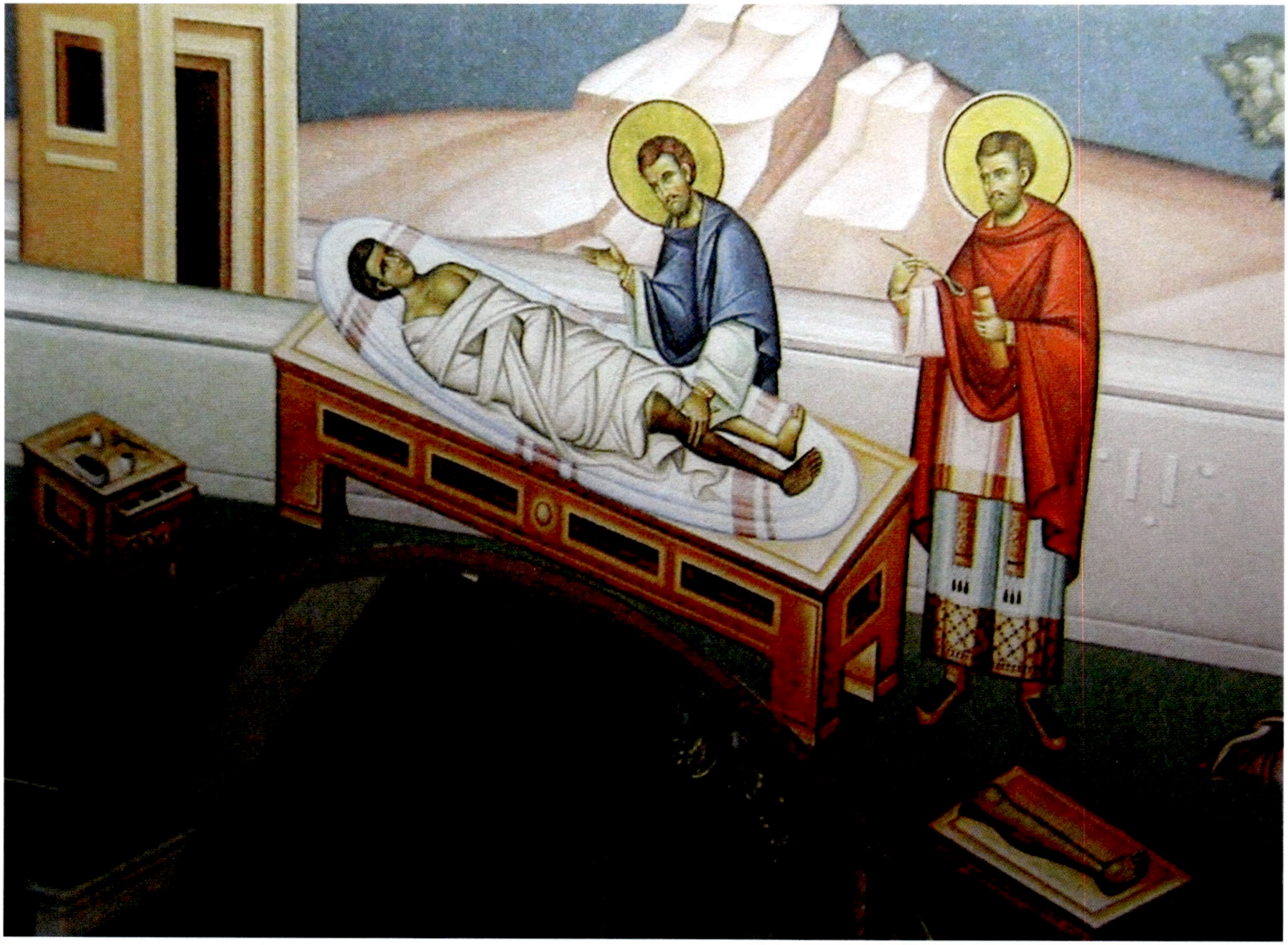

81. Stravos Gospodinis, *wallpainting,* 21th century. Ανάργυροι, Επταπύργιο (Church SS. Anargyri, Eptapyrgio), Thessaloniki (Greece).

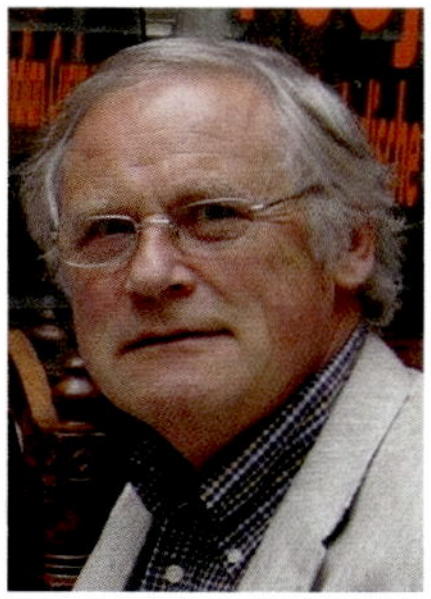

Kees Wouter Zimmerman has until his retirement in 2004 practiced as a trauma surgeon in the University Medical Centre of Groningen (UMCG). Within the traumatology he has among other subjects specialized in, and published on, operatic reconstruction of amputation stumps. It is no coincidence that this super-specialization led to his particular interest in the miracle of the transplantation of a leg by the saints Cosmas and Damian. Ever since 1987 Zimmerman has been collecting representations in art of the miracle performed by those saints . When he had collected 40 representations, this resulted in the publication of a book. This book, with the title "One Leg in the Grave" was published in 1998, at the occasion of the ninth World Congress of the International Society for Prosthesis and Orthotics (ISPO), in Amsterdam.

After his retirement, Zimmerman continued collecting representations of the miracle of the transplantation of the black leg.

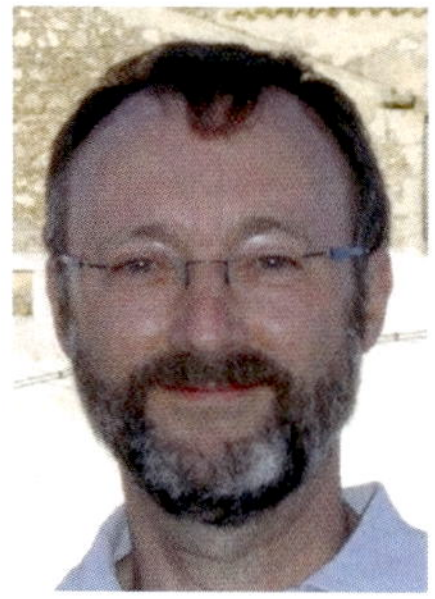

Jan L. de Jong studied art history at Leiden University, where he also wrote his Ph.D., on the interpretation of themes from classical mythology in Italian Renaissance painting, particularly in Roman palaces. Since then, he has focused on papal propaganda in painting. He has a book on this topic set for publication in 2013, at Penn State University Press. He is now working on Arnoldus Buchellius's *Iter Italicum*, from 1587. Jan de Jong is senior Lecture of Italian Renaissance Art at Groningen University, The Netherlands.

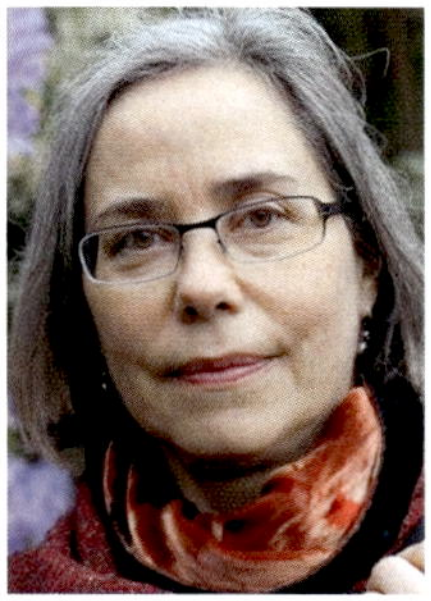

Carmen Fracchia is a Lecturer in Early Modern Spanish Art History at Birkbeck, University of London. She specializes in relations between the visual production and the formation of the Spanish Empire, with particular emphasis on visuality and slavery. She has been part of three international collaborative projects on Slavery and Abolition (2008-2013) at the University of Granada, Spain and she is currently writing a book-length project Black but Human: *Slavery and Visual Culture in Imperial Spain.*

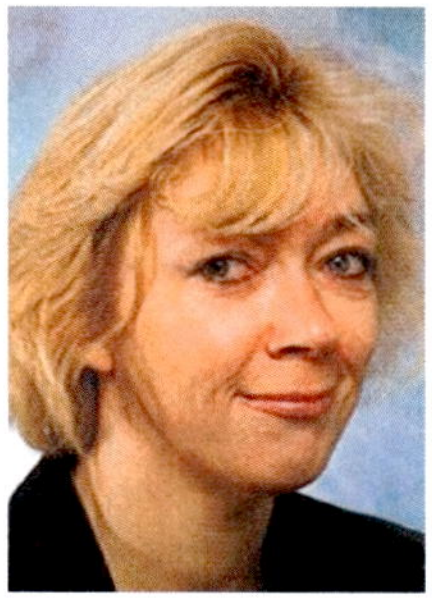

Catrien Santing studied history and art history at the University of Groningen. Between 1998 and 2003 she worked for the Dutch Institute in Rome. She is a cultural historian specialized in the Late Middle Ages and Renaissance. She focuses on the history of medicine and the body in the Late Middle Ages. Next to that she has widely published on Northern Humanism, Visual Culture, Medievalism and the Interchange between Art and Science. Currently she holds the chair of medieval history at the University of Groningen.

19W31431/ T1/ 97894914312341